COGNITIVE TECHNOLOGY IN PSYCHIATRIC REHABILITATION

Cognitive Technology

in Psychiatric Rehabilitation

William D. Spaulding

EDITOR

UNIVERSITY OF NEBRASKA PRESS

LINCOLN & LONDON

Manufactured in the United States of America.

The paper in this book meets the minimum requirements of American National Standard for Information Sciences – Permanence of Paper for Printed Library Materials, ANSI Z39.48-1984.

Library of Congress Cataloging-in-Publication Data
Cognitive technology in psychiatric rehabilitation / edited by William D. Spaulding. p. cm.
Includes bibliographical references and index.
ISBN 0-8032-4224-7 (cl.: alk. paper)
1. Mentally ill – Rehabilitation. 2. Cognition disorders – Patients – Rehabilitation. 3. Chronically ill – Rehabilitation. 4. Schizophrenics – Rehabilitation. 5. Mentally ill – Rehabilitation – Government policy. 6. Cognition disorders – Patients – Rehabilitation – Government policy.
I. Spaulding, William D. (William Delbert), 1950– .
[DNLM: 1. Psychotic Disorders – rehabilitation.
2. Cognition Disorders – rehabilitation.
3. Rehabilitation – methods. 4. Community Mental Health Services. WM 202 C676 1994]
RC439.5.C64 1994 616.89'1 – dc20 93-23685
DNLM/DLC for Library of Congress
CIP

This volume is dedicated to the memory of Werner Max Mendel, MD, formerly clinical director of Hastings (Nebraska) Regional Center and professor of psychiatry, University of Nebraska Medical Center. In the course of his brilliant career at the University of Southern California and later at Nebraska, Dr. Mendel wrote many articles and several books on schizophrenia. He was one of the original members of the group that collaborated to produce this volume, and he participated until his sudden death in 1990. He was a co-investigator with Robert Schalock in a statewide study of cognitive assessment and service planning.

CONTENTS

ILLUSTRATIONS

Figures

Tables

ACKNOWLEDGMENTS

A number of researchers, clinicians and administrators made important contributions to development of this volume, through participation in the cognitive technology conference and through their continuing interest in improving mental health services. To these individuals, grateful acknowledgment is made. They include Rue Cromwell, Patrick Corrigan, George Hannigan, Steve Higgins, Debra Hope, Glenda Housel, David Johnson, Bill Reay, Charles E. Richardson, Bill Shuart, and Martin Weiler. Acknowledgment is also made to the Nebraska Department of Public Institutions, whose generous support of various scholarly activities made this volume possible. Grateful acknowledgement is also made to Norma Jean Green for her dutiful secretarial help in preparing the manuscripts.

Introduction

The psychiatric research community has long accepted that impairments in cognitive functioning are associated with many severe and persistent psychiatric conditions, including schizophrenia, affective disorders, alcoholism, and others. Cognitive functioning here means the processes of sensation, perception, attention, conceptualization, problem solving, planning, and behavioral organization that are necessary to carry out routine personal and social activities.

Emil Kraepelin, who is usually credited with ushering in the contemporary era of psychiatry with his 1899 textbook of psychiatry (Kraepelin, 1899), used the concept of intellectual deterioration as a key characteristic in diagnosing schizophrenia, which was then called dementia praecox. Intellectual functioning is rather rudimentary as a cognitive construct, but Kraepelin's recognition that insanity represents more than perverse motivations and preoccupations, being associated in fact with disruption of normal brain functions, was a landmark in the history of psychopathology.

The first half of the twentieth century saw voluminous theorizing and a fair amount of empirical research on cognitive deficits in psychiatric disorders. Because much of this work stemmed from psychoanalytic theory, its focus was on developmental psychosexual and psychosocial processes that were hypothesized to produce the deficits. The pinnacle of this work is Arieti's (1955) theory of schizophrenia, in which various psychodynamic factors operate to induce use of paleologic instead of normal adult logic. Paleologic is a primitive form that fails grammatically to distinguish predicate from subject. Hence, in paleologic, one might think, 'Gorillas have hair, I have hair, therefore I am a gorilla.' Arieti reasoned that the schizophrenic patient's cognitive functioning regresses to a childlike state, in which this type of logic is developmentally normal. Following the revered biological principle that ontogeny recapitulates phylogeny, he further hypothesized that a child's logic is structurally similar to the logic that was used by protohuman species, hence the name paleologic. Many of the linguistic and behavioral abnormalities of schizophrenia can be understood as following from the patient's use of this type of faulty thinking.

Arieti's theory was an elegant integration of psychoanalytic principles, descriptive clinical psychiatry, and the cognitive psychology of his era. Unfortunately, it did not survive, for a number of reasons. For one, the accumulating evidence of congenital and genetic factors in schizophrenia casts serious doubt on any theory that relies solely on experiential etiological factors, as is the case with psychoanalytic theories. Nor did the theory lead to significant changes in the psychoanalytic approach to treatment of schizophrenia. There is no experimental evidence that the processes described by Arieti could be reversed to cure the patient.

Another reason for the demise of Arieti's model came from developments in cognitive psychopathology. In the 1930s David Shakow, later one of the founding figures of American clinical psychology, began his research on schizophrenia by setting up a psychology laboratory at Worcester Hospital in Massachusetts. Using the standard psychological measurement paradigms of his day, ranging from intelligence tests to reaction time measures, Shakow articulated the cognitive impairments of schizophrenia in more precise and quantified terms than had been achieved before. Among other things, Shakow's work (1977) clearly showed that the impairments extend to the most basic psychological functions, such as attention and memory. This depth of impairment makes it difficult to argue that the source of all schizophrenic abnormalities lies at a high and complex level of cognition, such as logical processing. How could failure of logic disrupt simple reaction time?

Progress in all aspects of psychopathology was slowed during the 1950s by confusion about the validity of psychiatric diagnosis. It is impossible to compare diagnostic categories of patients meaningfully if the criteria for categorization are themselves problematic. This difficulty was compounded by psychopathologists' assumption that they were looking for a single "key" deficit of schizophrenia, a search later compared by Cromwell (1984) to the quest for the Holy Grail. Gradually, the realization grew that "diseases" such as schizophrenia are actually groups or families of symptom syndromes, not necessarily related to each other through common etiological processes. Similarly, it became clear that there is no "one true deficit" at the root of schizophrenia or related disorders. Patients who fit even the modern diagnostic criteria have individually unique constellations of cognitive deficits.

In the 1970s schizophrenia and other severe psychiatric disorders began to attract the attention of clinical neuropsychologists. Originating in neurosurgery services, clinical neuropsychology had been enormously successful in using cognitive measures to localize anatomically discrete brain lesions and to characterize their functional effects. Ironically, it was initially considered disappointing that neuropsychological tests proved unable to distinguish chronic brain injury from chronic schizophrenia. As evidence accumulated for neurobiological factors in schizophrenia, this view of things was turned on its head and researchers began to hypothesize that chronic schizophrenia is, among other things, the result of brain injury of various kinds. Today, experimental psychopathology, neuropathology, and neuropsychology have begun to converge. Current theories of severe psychiatric disorders address not only the precise nature of cognitive deficits, but also the brain structures in which lesions or functional abnormalities might produce such deficits, as well as the etiological processes that might produce the lesions.

There are still disagreements about how various cognitive and/or neuropsychological impairments are related to the primary causes of various disorders, but there is no disagreement that once cognitive impairments appear, they are significant handicaps that interfere with recovery and rehabilitation. Lingering cognitive impairments are seen by many rehabilitation professionals as the major obstacles to achieving gainful employment, independent living, and the quality of life those achievements confer.

The importance of cognitive functioning has been highlighted in the development over the past decade of psychiatric rehabilitation. Psychiatric rehabilitation is a multimodal, multidisciplinary approach grounded in principles that evolved from rehabilitation psychology, occupational therapy, and physical medicine. In addition to receiving standard pharmacological and behavioral treatment, patients are trained or retrained in the skills necessary for the routines of independent living and for social and personal functioning, e.g., housekeeping, hygienic self-care, social skills, medication self-management, and emotional self-regulation. Patients' cognitive functioning may determine to a significant degree how much they benefit from these skill-training activities, and thus how much independent functioning they ultimately regain. Similarly, patients' level of cognitive functioning may determine what level of community services they need, e.g., whether they can live in their own apartments or whether they require a more highly structured community residential facility. Stated in the most general terms, cognitive impairments limit the effectiveness of almost all the treatment (even drug treatment), rehabilitation, and social services available to those who are impaired.

There are many instruments and methods by which to assess cognitive functioning, but most are not especially well suited to the special problems and needs of the severely and persistently disordered. The recent scientific and technological developments that have more potential are not used with any uniformity or consistency in mental health systems. Efficient use of information about patients' cognitive functioning may require system-wide acceptance of a set of instruments and measures to be used uniformly throughout the service system.

Recently, developments in several clinical research domains have begun to converge on the possibility of directly treating cognitive deficits. This approach has been inspired in part by a growing realization that neuroleptic drugs are remarkably limited in their ability to normalize cognitive functioning in schizophrenia beyond suppression of the most disruptive symptoms characteristic of the acute phase of the disorder. Well-controlled studies to confirm the clinical potential of direct cognitive treatment are beginning to appear. As with assessment techniques, the treatment approaches have grown from diverse scientific disciplines and clinical professional communities.

There is thus a growing sense that cognitive technologies for psychiatric rehabilitation should be developed and introduced into mental health systems. In response, this volume is a compendium of theory and research from pioneers in relevant areas. In addition to evaluating the scientific and technological validity of cognitive approaches, the contributors to this volume identify basic issues and considerations for introducing new technologies into mental health service systems. This is a domain of historic failures. If they are to be effective, cognitive technologies may require fundamental changes in service systems and even in professional training programs, given the nature of cognitive technology, the nature of psychiatric rehabilitation, and the universal characteristics of mental health systems. It is hoped that this volume will facilitate eventual use of the technology it promulgates by informing clinicians, administrators, and researchers about general and specific implementation issues.

This volume is divided into three parts. The four chapters in the first part emphasize clinical assessment issues. In the first chapter, Claudia Allen discusses cognitive assessment for psychiatric rehabilitation from the perspective of occupational therapy. Her approach identifies levels of cognitive impairment with functional limitations on patients' abilities to engage in normal occupations and activities. Similar functional approaches have been successful in rehabilitation of physical disabilities. Allen argues that such approaches are not only useful for treatment and dispositional planning but in fact necessary for accountable administration and provision of rehabilitation services. Students and professionals in occupational therapy will find in this chapter an application of familiar tools and principles to clinical problems that may be unfamiliar. Readers from other disciplines will find a brief but enlightening introduction to occupational therapy perspectives on assessment, rehabilitation, and health care policy.

The next chapter, by Robert Schalock and Werner Mendel, is a companion piece to Allen's chapter. It is an empirical analysis of Allen's cognitive assessment system, using what is possibly the largest sample ever constructed of longitudinal assessment data on cognitive functioning in chronic substance abuse and psychiatric patients. In the third chapter, Richard Erickson describes a comprehensive model for systematic assessment and service planning using the cognitive technology of clinical neuropsychology. Finally, Robert Kern and Michael Green describe a research program that articulates some of the specific consequences of cognitive impairment in rehabilitation modalities.

Together, these first four chapters present alternative but not incompatible theoretical conceptualizations of cognitive assessment in service planning, as well as initial empirical data on its use and effectiveness. There are many purposes to which clinical assessment may be put, in mental health generally and in rehabilitation particularly. No single instrument, not even a single general approach, can be expected to meet all needs. Among the diverse approaches described in this section, each is probably better suited to some applications than others. For example, straightforward functional models and easy-to-administer instruments like those in Allen's approach may commend it to large-scale policy, system planning, and administrative applications, while the fine-grained specificity of neuropsychological assessment is most useful in treatment of the individual patient.

The five chapters in the second part concern direct treatment of cognitive impairments. All five include theoretical conceptualization, descriptions of actual service programs that use cognitive principles, and empirical outcome data. Joel Goldberg describes a rehabilitation program, based on a neuropsychological model, that emphasizes treatment of the more molecular deficits (attention, memory, etc.) of schizophrenia. Susan Fine describes a program with similar goals that takes the perspective of occupational therapy: it makes extensive use of commercially available computer-video technology.

Fine also discusses the relationship of her program to the governmental and social policy climate of the state of New York. Martin Appelo and his colleagues describe a comprehensive approach to rehabilitation, built on models of social learning and cognition and sensitive to social policy as seen from a European perspective. Mark van der Gaag elaborates on the cognitive treatment component of this program, presenting detailed information on its effectiveness. Finally, Robert Heinssen describes a rehabilitation program in which the cognitive orientation comes from yet another clinical tradition, that of cognitive-behavioral psychotherapy.

While all of these chapters touch on issues of technology implementation, the three chapters in the third part of this volume focus on mental health systems issues rather than the technology itself. Mark DeKraai and Peter Beeson discuss considerations for introducing new technologies from the perspective of mental health system planning and administration. Peter Magaro, who discusses the historical context of innovation in mental health services, issues important warnings about unreflective adoption of technological models. Mary Sullivan describes the interactions of researchers (including contributors to this volume and others), clinicians, and administrators at a special conference on cognitive technology in psychiatric rehabilitation, held at the University of Nebraska–Lincoln in 1991. These three chapters, together with the preceding ones, create an extensive map of the issues and obstacles to be expected in professional and scientific communities when introducing cognitive technology into current service systems.

References

Arieti, S. (1955). *Interpretation of schizophrenia.* New York: Bruner-Mazel.

Cromwell, R. (1984). Preemptive thinking and schizophrenia research. In W. Spaulding and J. Cole (Eds.), *Nebraska Symposium on Motivation,* Vol. 31*: Theories of Schizophrenia and Psychosis.* Lincoln: University of Nebraska Press.

Kraepelin, E. (1899). *Psychiatrie: Ein Lehrbuch für studirende und Ärzte.* Leipzig: Verlag von Johann Ambrosius Barth.

Shakow, D. (1977). *Schizophrenia: Collected papers.* New York: International Universities Press.

• 1 •

Functional Outcomes of Physical and Psychosocial Rehabilitation

Claudia Kay Allen

Medicine and rehabilitation deal with different kinds of problems and produce different kinds of outcomes. Medicine is driven by the cause of a disease and is expected to prevent or reverse that cause. Rehabilitation is driven by the consequences of health problems that cannot be prevented or cured. Its objective is to maximize the individual's remaining ability to function (Allen & Mendel, 1982). The expected outcome is optimal adjustment of patients, families, and other people in the support system to the realities of living with residual disabilities. Thus, in contrast to the curative outcome expected in medicine, the goal of rehabilitation is a functional outcome.

There are important differences between a psychiatric and a physical disability in terms of adjustment. A physical disability is usually quite evident to the patient and others. Psychiatric disabilities are often cognitive impairments, resulting from brain pathology, that can be overlooked or excused, sometimes until the patient engages in unacceptable or dangerous behavior. Nevertheless, cognitive disabilities may have serious effects, however subtle, on many of a patient's activities, which may require considerable readjustment on the part of patients and their community support systems. Failure to understand impairment of cognitive abilities often results in failures in adjustment, a pattern that in turn leads to blaming the patient for lack of motivation. When a patient cannot respond to expectations because of brain pathology, part of the process of rehabilitation is helping people understand the difference between "will not" and "cannot."

Most people experience a cognitive disability at some point during their lifetimes, usually in response to fever or fatigue. Temporary cognitive disabilities are of little social consequence because social allowances are made for them. We adapt by taking some aspirin, going to bed, taking time off from work, and avoiding demanding or dangerous situations. Disabilities that extend beyond the usual social allowances, like two weeks of sick time, require more social support. The long-term disabilities associated with severe psychiatric disorders require much more allowance and support, of course. Unfortunately, people seldom have a natural understanding of the implications of cognitive disabilities based on their own experience. It usually falls to the clinician to help patients and their caregivers develop such an understanding.

This chapter describes an approach to evaluating cognitive disabilities in the context of psychiatric rehabilitation. Although the approach was developed from the perspective of occupational therapy, its usefulness is not necessarily limited to that discipline. Similarly, although its development was based on experience with psychiatric patients, the approach is potentially applicable also to patients whose disabilities have other origins. The primary purpose of evaluation in this approach is to determine the kinds of activities or occupations in which a patient with cognitive disabilities can safely engage. This determination has direct consequences for the care setting that the patient requires, and to some degree for the strategy of the patient's rehabilitation.

Defining Cognitive and Occupational Disabilities

The origins of brain pathology are important in other contexts, but in rehabilitation the focus is on how brain pathology affects a patient's performance of activities. In this case, the distinction between psychiatric and neurological disorders is artificial. Rehabilitation must address cognitive disabilities whether their origins are psychiatric or neurological. (However, the origins of the pathology may influence the age at which disabilities appear, and the timing has important implications for rehabilitation. Children who have not acquired extensive activity repertoires present a different problem than adults, even though the adult may have lost much of what has already been learned.) For this reason, rehabilitation terminology must identify relevant disabilities independent of their origin, i.e., independent of the psychiatric or neurological diagnosis. The International Classification of Impairments, Disabilities and Handicaps (ICIDH; World Health Organization, 1980) describes a cognitive disability as one that restricts a person's ability to engage in customary occupations. Such activities include "routine tasks, school, work, play/leisure, and social activities according to ordinary community standards for the quality of performance and the time scheduled for doing these activities" (p.195). In this terminology, rehabilitation services produce an optimal outcome by maximizing a disabled individual's opportunities to engage in customary occupations.

The ICIDH definition identifies cognitive disabilities as a legitimate area of concern for occupational therapists and other professionals. For the purposes of clinical evaluation and treatment planning, however, a more extensive and detailed terminology is required. A terminological system for classifying cognitive disabilities has been developed over a number of years (Allen, 1982, 1985, 1988; Allen & Allen, 1987). The system has recently been codified in the *Medicare Intermediary Manual,* part 3 (Health Care Financing Administration, 1990), a document that has become important for administrative classification of patients who need nursing and other health care.

The Allen system defines cognitive disability in terms of six levels, ranging from profound disability at level 1 to normal ability at level 6. Each cognitive level is associated with the level of assistance needed, from total assistance to independent status. Assistance is defined in terms of the social conditions that must be in place to maximize abilities safely. A need for greater sensitivity has led to subdivisions within the levels, describing 52 modes of performance (Allen, Earhart & Blue, 1992), which are beyond the scope of this chapter.

At level 1, people are usually confined to hospital beds with the side rails up to prevent falling. Responses to stimuli indicate that they are conscious. Nourishment is provided intravenously or in the form of pureed food that is fed or eaten using a cup and a spoon. Twenty-four-hour nursing care is required to maintain skin integrity by preventing bedsores and by bathing and cleaning after voiding.

At level 2, people are able to overcome gravity by sitting up. Other gross body movements include righting reactions, aimless or directed walking, and using "grab bars" for postural stability. Twenty-four-hour nursing care is required to provide food, to initiate and guide use of the toilet and bath, to prevent wandering, to point out stairs or uneven surfaces, and to make sure that grab bars, rails, and furniture are stable.

At level 3, people use their hands to manipulate objects. Manual actions include grasp and release, motions appropriate in handling familiar objects like a hairbrush or a toothbrush, and other repetitive actions, and people at level 3 take note of the effects of such actions. Twenty-four-hour supervision is required to maintain an acceptable level of hygiene, to ensure completion of the steps of self-care activities, and to prevent access to dangerous objects and situations.

At level 4, people can guide themselves through the steps of routine activities such as self-care and other daily chores. Memories of how to carry out frequently performed activities are grossly intact, as are vocabulary, arithmetic, and social manners. It is when something out of the ordinary happens, requiring the translation of new information into modified motor actions, that the cognitive disability becomes apparent. Daily assistance is required to solve minor problems, to prevent access to dangerous objects and situations, and to provide an allowance of money, as well as reminders of household chores and community events to be attended.

Learning an activity by doing occurs at level 5. Variations in neuromuscular actions are explored in terms of the effects they have on objects. People at this level can learn the primary effects of their actions but cannot anticipate the secondary effects. Problems with judgment, impulse control, and selfishness are common and are often labeled "personality disorders" in mental health settings. Supervision is required to point out the potential for accidents and to make sure that safety precautions are followed consistently. Restricted access to risky materials like power tools and combustibles is recommended.

At level 6, unwanted secondary effects of actions are anticipated and avoided. A plan of action is premeditated before any action is started, and actions can be adjusted during the process of performing an activity. Several hypothetical plans can be considered simultaneously, and deductive reasoning employed to select the best plan. The individual is independent in making plans for the future that take into account risks to the health and well-being of self and others.

Assessment methods and instruments

In most psychiatric settings, the most immediately relevant assessment question is whether a patient is functioning at level 3, 4, or 5. The answer requires an assessment of a broad range of the patient's activities. The problem in evaluating human activities is that there are so many of them. Occupational therapists use a system of activity analysis to evaluate the cognitive complexity of major roles and spare-time activities. Considerable observation in both natural and structured settings is required.

In determining a patient's level of cognitive functioning, it is important to consider both the ability and the motivation to perform certain activities. Performance of an activity that the patient finds uninteresting or unmotivating may not represent a valid picture of the patient's cognitive abilities. The clinician must be prepared to assess performance ability in any activity toward which the patient is motivationally inclined. For patients who are not motivated to engage in many activities, evaluation is difficult. The handicraft activities familiar to most occupational therapists are advantageous in this regard, being intrinsically interesting or motivating for most people and providing good opportunities for observation. For patients whose motivation or interests are extremely limited, criteria are available for estimating the cognitive complexity of virtually any legal activity (Allen, 1985; Allen, Earhart & Blue, 1992). Most patients at level 3 or above can be clinically assessed by using these criteria to evaluate the complexity of whatever activity the patient chooses.

Despite the necessity of both natural and structured settings, some standardized assessments can be useful for clinical and research purposes.

The Allen Cognitive Level (ACL) Test is a screening tool for quickly assessing levels 3, 4, and 5. The patient is asked to imitate three leather lacing stitches: a sewing, a whip, and a single cordovan stitch. Each stitch is done three times or until patients make an error that they cannot correct. The ACL has been around long enough that several versions have been developed. The original was published in 1985 (Allen). Later research studies (Mayer, 1988; Newman, 1987; Earhart & Allen, 1988) prompted an expansion of the scoring scale, which, among other things, now allows comparison with Wechsler intelligence scales (Mayer, 1988). The relationships with other common measures of psychopathology were investigated by David & Riley (1990). Visual impairments that interfere with seeing the leather stitches prompted development of a physically larger version (Allen, Earhart & Blue, 1992). Problems with a capping effect, plus difficulties in making clear separations within levels 5 and 6, prompted a new method of giving the instructions (Josman & Katz, 1991). Cross-cultural studies are beginning to examine the universal nature of the cognitive levels (Katz & Heimann, 1990; Cusick & Harai, 1991). A kit and testing manual for the 1990 version of the ACL are commercially available. The ease of administration and scoring has made the ACL a popular clinical and research tool.

The Routine Task Inventory (RTI) utilizes functional descriptions of behavior associated with each of the six cognitive levels. The original list of self-care and instrumental activities of daily living was taken from an inventory developed by Lawton and Brody (1969). Reliability and validity data are available for the original list of activities, based on caregiver reports (Heinmann, Allen & Yerxa, 1989; Wilson et al., 1989). An expanded version of the RTI is also available (Earhart & Allen, 1988). Two subscales for communication and work/leisure were added, with an analysis for child care and therapeutic exercise. Occupational role and social role activities have recently been added (Allen, Earhart & Blue, 1992). Work on developing a standardized performance test based on RTI descriptions has been started by Burns (Allen, Earhart & Blue, 1992).

Additional activities for standardized assessments have been investigated, but as a whole less is known about their reliability and validity as measurements. A scratch pad assembly task was standardized for the first study done by Herzig (Allen, 1985) and was found to correlate ($r = .73$) with the ACL (Richards, 1983). Standardized procedures for checking safety awareness while cooking are available for people functioning at level 4. The tasks include making pudding and a macaroni and cheese dish. A relationship was found between the ACL score and the number of errors made while preparing macaroni and cheese (Alsberg, 1987).

Assessed Cognitive Level, Postacute Care and Rehabilitation

Referral for postacute care is an occasion for assessment of patients' cognitive levels. Acute psychotic episodes or relapses usually necessitate hospitalization for periods of several days to several months. During this period, as the psychotic condition restabilizes in response to antipsychotic drugs and the hospital milieu, some improvement in cognitive level is expected. As cognitive level reaches a plateau, it becomes relevant to considerations about the patient's postacute care needs. The primary consideration is the least restrictive environment in which the patient can function safely at the time of discharge. Discharge recommendations should take cognitive level into account and should include, for example, warnings about safety hazards that may not be noticed by the patient, suggested changes in the home or work environment that may protect people from injury or prevent property damage, recommendations for changes in legal status when patients are unable to manage their own affairs, and suggestions for rehabilitation services (Allen, Earhart & Blue, 1992).

In psychiatric rehabilitation, the patient engages in many different activities, for a variety of purposes. The specific regimen of activities included in a rehabilitation plan takes into account the patient's history and preferences, the physical and social environment in which the patient is to function, the availability and characteristics of caregivers, rehabilitation goals, and the patient's cognitive level.

As with postacute care planning, a primary consideration is the patient's safety. Some rehabilitation activities may expose the patient to situations that are hazardous because of the patient's cognitive level. The potential value of an activity must be weighed against such hazards. Sometimes potentially helpful activities must be postponed or even forgone because of overriding safety considerations.

One important focus of rehabilitation is to reestablish basic activities that have been lost in the course of the disorder, most often the routines of daily living such as hygiene and self-care. The occupational therapist promotes reestablishment of these abilities through structured, repetitive drilling, preferably in settings and circumstances identical to those in which the activities are normally completed. The length of training time required to drill in a new skill depends on the availability of memories of how to perform similar activities. Availability of such memories is usually reflected in the patient's cognitive level; lower levels are associated with fewer available memories. For all but the highest cognitive levels, generalization is a problem in reestablishing abilities. That is, even when an activity can be reliably performed in a particular setting under supervision of the therapist, slightly different circumstances may prevent performance. Additional drilling in the new setting may be necessary, and in some cases the only solution may be to provide continuing supervision in new settings.

Medicare, as well as most insurance policies, excludes repetitive drilling from rehabilitation services (Health Care Financing Administration, 1990). The patient's caregiver thus becomes responsible for conducting and/or supervising therapeutic activities, and the professional therapist must plan for this eventuality in most rehabilitation programs. Teaching and training thus become an important part of the therapist's role. The implications of a patient's cognitive disabilities, as well as other functional limitations, must be explained. Drilling procedures must be demonstrated. The implications for patient safety must be reviewed. The continuing success of rehabilitation may be heavily dependent on the therapist's skill in imparting this understanding to nonprofessional caregivers.

As in the case of physical disabilities, patients and their caregivers must come to terms emotionally and psychologically with the losses that their cognitive disabilities represent. Helping them do this is always part of the role of the therapist. Reactions may range from sanguine acceptance to assertive denial of disabilities. In some cases, denial can lead to dangerous circumstances, as when a patient insists on continuing to drive even though cognitive impairments make driving very dangerous. It is neither helpful nor responsible for the professional to accede to such a situation. Learning to live with limitations is an important part of rehabilitation, and the therapist must sometimes take difficult positions in acknowledging that reality. When necessary, therapists must be prepared to take steps to initiate legal action such as removing a driver's license or obtaining a legal guardian (Allen, Earhart & Blue, 1992).

Cognitive Level and Continuing Care

Rehabilitation is completed when all abilities that can be reestablished are in place, and when adjustment to residual disabilities is optimal. Even when rehabilitation is successful, the severity of residual disabilities and the assistance required to adjust to them may require the patient to remain in some type of care setting. This is as true for cognitive as for physical disabilities. It is at this point that continuing or long-term care must be provided. Without this service, the patient's behavior may deteriorate. Psychotic relapse and substance abuse may aggravate the deterioration, including deterioration of cognitive level. Ultimately the patient is in danger of becoming a homeless person, in failing physical and mental health.

Continuing care consists of providing an activity program for disabled people within an environment that ensures the safety of both the disabled and the community, while minimizing restrictiveness. The time over which this service must be provided is determined by the prognosis for continued participation in functional activities. The expected outcome is maintenance of remaining functional abilities within a supportive context and avoidance of secondary complications that could increase the health and social welfare demands.

To participate in such programs, people must be willing to accept other disabled and handicapped people as their peers. Control of drug and alcohol abuse as well as behavior that is dangerous to self and others must be ensured by the program or the patient. Activities that match the person's cognitive level can prevent the emergence of behaviors that might cause problems in less supportive settings. In the United States, certified occupational therapy assistants have the knowledge required to match the demands of an activity to a disabled person's remaining abilities.

Initially, the concerns in assessing the need for continuing care are generally the same as those for postacute care, except, of course, that they must be reevaluated in light of whatever changes take place in the course of rehabilitation. In the longer term, the assessment must address whether or not a care plan can do all the following in a way consonant with the patient's cognitive level:

1. Provide activities acceptable to the individual;
2. Recognize residual cognitive limitations that will require modification in the usual procedure if a task is to be performed successfully, and make the necessary modifications tactfully;
3. Replicate a sense of the individual's normal place in history and culture as closely as possible;
4. Replace deviant behavior with behavior that is socially acceptable;
5. Arrange for participation in normal community events whenever economically feasible and socially acceptable;
6. Arrange for access to social welfare and health care resources when needed;
7. Work with available social support systems to maintain the highest level of function by explaining the difference between "cannot" and "will not" to other people in the community;
8. Assist other caregivers in making environmental changes that either reduce the burden of care or improve functional abilities;
9. Facilitate departure from the long-term care system whenever permitted by changes in the disability or in social conditions (such as money for supportive employment).

A long-term care program is not transitional and people should be allowed to continue in it as long as they want to and need to do so. Very few people should be expected to resume an independent schedule of participation in normal community activities without special assistance. The most probable discharge criterion is that the condition will not worsen to an extent that prevents the individual from functioning.

Implications for Health Care Policy

Unfortunately, the deinstitutionalization movement of the past two decades has not led to better rehabilitation and continuing care services for people with cognitive disabilities. Hopefully, greater recognition of the similarities between cognitive and physical disability will help correct this situation. Under the new Americans with Disabilities Act, citizens are entitled to services for a disability when the disability is severe enough to prohibit participation in the usual community activities, given reasonable accommodation, and when there is a demonstrated need for the specialized knowledge of a therapist.

As a terminological system, the Allen Cognitive Levels should facilitate development of services for people with cognitive disabilities because the levels describe functional abilities and losses much as physical disabilites are described. It is fairly well established that service financing models can effectively be built around functional criteria for physical disabilities (Wilkerson, Batavia & DeJong, 1992). It is not yet clear how health care entitlements may apply to functionally defined cognitive disabilities, and there will likely be much discussion and debate about what constitutes "reasonable accommodation," especially for disabilities that allow the patient to function at cognitive level 4 or above (Allen, Earhart & Blue, 1992). In any case, however, use of functional criteria for cognitive disabilities demonstrates that the consequences of psychiatric and neurological disorders are equivalent, and understanding of this equivalence should help overcome the double standard of care for psychiatric and physical disabilities.

A similar advantage of functional terminology applies to assessment of service outcome. Outcome has become an important consideration in health care policy, and rehabilitation is no exception. Any service must show itself worthy of funding by demonstrating that it produces meaningful outcomes. In rehabilitation, such a demonstration has often been required on a case-by-case basis. At first, sheer objectivity in outcome measurement was thought to be the solution. During the 1970s and 1980s, physical rehabilitation therapists were required to identify and achieve measurable treatment objectives for each of their patients if they were to be reimbursed. The result was that therapists got very good at writing measurable objectives of questionable importance. To solve this problem, the insurance industry has shifted to requiring functional outcomes. For example, Blue Cross of California defines a functional outcome as meaningful, utilitarian, and sustainable. A meaningful ability is the capacity to do, safely and effectively, an activity that is valued by the patient and/or caregiver. Utilitarian performance is the most economical and efficient, and sustainable performance maintains its quality outside the clinical setting.

As health care costs continue to rise, the nation is moving in the direction of demanding an accountable and cost-effective health care system. The successful providers of rehabilitation services will be those who solve the problems of individual patients at a reasonable cost. Psychiatric and psychosocial rehabilitation must work within those constraints.

References

Allen, C. K. (1982). Independence through activity: The practice of occupational therapy (psychiatry). *American Journal of Occupational Therapy,* 36, 731–739.

Allen, C. K. (1985). *Occupational therapy for psychiatric diseases: Measurement and management of cognitive disabilities.* Boston: Little, Brown and Co.

Allen, C. K. (1987a). Occupational therapy: Measuring the severity of mental disorders. *Hospital and Community Psychiatry* 38:140–142.

Allen, C. K. (1987b). Activity: Occupational therapy's treatment method (Eleanor Clarke Slagle Lecture—1987). *American Journal of Occupational Therapy,* 41, 563–575.

Allen, C. K. (1988). Cognitive disabilities. In S. Robinson (Ed.). *Focus.* Rockville, Md.: American Occupational Therapy Association.

Allen, C. K. (1989). Treatment plans in cognitive rehabilitation. *Occupational Therapy Practice,* 1, 1–8.

Allen, C. K. (1990). *Allen Cognitive Level Test manual* (including kit). Coldchester, Conn.: S&S/Worldwide.

Allen, C. K., & Allen, R. E. (1987). Cognitive disabilities: Measuring the social consequences of mental disorders. *Journal of Clinical Psychiatry,* 48, 185–191.

Allen, C. K., Earhart, C. A., & Blue, T. (1992). Occupational therapy treatment goals for the physically and cognitively disabled. Rockville, Md.: American Occupational Therapy Association.

Allen, C. K., & Mendel, W. M. (1982). Chronic illness and staff burn-out: Revised expectations for change in the supportive-care model. *International Journal of Partial Hospitalization,* 1, 191–201.

Alsberg, D. (1987). Safety implications of cognitive disabilities: Using cognitive theory as an adjunct to discharge planning. Unpublished master's thesis, Rush University.

American Psychiatric Association. (1987). *Diagnostic and statistical manual.* 3rd Edition. Revised. Washington, D.C.: American Psychiatric Association.

Cusick, A., & Harai, H. (1991). The Allen tests for cognitive disability: A cross cultural pilot study. *Occupational Therapy in Mental Health,* 11, 61–75.

David, S. K., & Riley, W. T. (1989). The relationship of the Allen Cognitive Level Test to cognitive abilities and psychopathology. *American Journal of Occupational Therapy,* 44, 493–497.

Earhart, C. A., & Allen, C. K. (1988). Cognitive disabilities: Expanded activity analysis. Colchester, Conn.: S&S/Worldwide.

Gilinsky, A. S. (1984). *Mind and brain: Principles of neuropsychology.* New York: Praeger.

Health Care Financing Administration (1990). *Medicare intermediary manual,* part 3; claims processing transmittal no. 1487, section 3906 (Sept. 1990). Baltimore: Health Care Financing Administration.

Heimann, N. E., Allen, C. K., & Yerxa, E. J. (1989). The routine task inventory: a tool for describing the functional behavior of the cognitively disabled. *Occupational Therapy Practice,* 1, 67–74.

Josman, N., & Katz, N. (1991). Problem solving version of the Allen Cognitive Level (ACL) test. *American Journal of Occupational Therapy,* 45, 331–338.

Katz, N., & Heimann, N. (1990). Review of research conducted in Israel on cognitive disability instrumentation. *Occupational Therapy in Mental Health,* 10, 1–15.

Lawton, M. P., & Brody, E.M. (1969). Assessment of older people: Self-maintaining and instrumental activities of daily living. *Gerontologist,* 9, 179–186.

Mayer, M. A. (1988). Analysis of information processing and cognitive disability theory. *American Journal of Occupational Therapy,* 42, 176–183.

Miller, R. (1981). *Meaning and purpose in the intact brain: A philosophical, psychological, and biological account of conscious processes.* New York: Clarendon Press.

Newman, M. (1987). Cognitive disability and functional performance in individuals with chronic schizophrenic disorders. Master's Thesis, University of Southern California.

Richards, G. E. (1983). Evaluation of the Allen Cognitive Level Test as an occupational therapy assessment tool. Unpublished master's thesis, West Chester State College.

Wilkerson, D. L., Batavia, A. I., & DeJong, G. (1992). Use of functional status measures for payment of medical rehabilitation services. *Archives of Physical Medicine and Rehabilitation,* 73, 111–119.

Wilson, D. S., Allen, C. K., McCormack, G., & Burton, G. (1989). Cognitive disability and routine task behaviors in a community based population with senile dementia. *Occupational Therapy Practice,* 1, 58–66.

World Health Organization (1980). International classification of impairments, disabilities, and handicaps. Geneva, Switzerland: WHO.

• 2 •

Assessment of Cognitive Level in Mental Health Systems

Robert L. Schalock

This chapter focuses on two issues in cognitive and behavioral rehabilitation. One issue is the relationship of cognitive functioning to rehabilitation outcome in psychiatric patients; the second is the relevance of cognitive level to behavioral changes as they develop over time. Throughout this chapter, cognitive functioning is discussed in terms of "cognitive level," operationalized as scores obtained from the Allen Cognitive Level Test (Allen, 1986).

Cognitive Level and Outcomes in Psychiatric Patients

The effectiveness of most psychiatric treatment is controversial and equivocal. To date, research on psychiatric outcomes has used a number of outcome variables, including hospital recidivism, duration of out-of-hospital time, vocational and recreational activities, degree of social adjustment, and level of current symptoms. Recidivism has been the most frequently used outcome variable. Identification of patient characteristics that differentially predict outcome has also been problematic. With the exception of the number of previous admissions, few consistent predictors of rehospitalization have been reported (Anthony, Cohen & Vitalo, 1978; Franklin, Kittridge & Thrasher, 1975; Lambert, Sherwood & Fitzpatrick, 1983; Rosenblatt & Mayer, 1974). A recent review of studies of social, social-psychological, and psychiatric correlates of community adaptation among psychiatric patients concluded that

The author is indebted to the late Dr. Werner Max Mendel for his conceptualization and support of the work summarized in this article. Appreciation is also expressed to Michael Sheehan for his administrative support, and to Linda Weber and Ruby Adler for their technical assistance.

over the past decade, little theoretical or methodological progress has been made in identifying factors conducive to patients' successful community adjustment (Avison & Speechley, 1987). One reason for this lack of progress is that researchers do not often use multiple predictor variables and multivariate analyses for model development and hypothesis testing (Bartko, Carpenter & McGlashan, 1988; Goering et al., 1984; Lambert et al., 1983; Miller, Beck & Fraps, 1984; Wright et al., 1989).

Assessed cognitive level has been one of several predictor variables evaluated during the last three years in an ongoing multivariate study at Hastings Regional Center (HRC), a state mental hospital in central Nebraska. The study has attempted to determine what factors influence the posthospital course of psychiatric patients. Every second patient admitted to the Psychiatric Unit is selected for study. Interview and record review data are collected at three points: at admission, discharge, and 12 months following discharge. Data presented in this chapter came from 267 subjects. Major diagnostic groups include organic brain syndrome (7.6% of the sample), schizophrenic disorders (35%), other psychiatric disorders (8.5%), affective disorders (25.6%), and adjustment disorders (9.4%). Details of study procedures are described in the *Management Study Manual* (Schalock, 1988).

The primary outcome variable in the study is recidivism, which is defined as returned to HRC or any other state-administered psychiatric facility within 12 months following discharge. Thirty-two predictor variables corresponding to prehospital, in-hospital, and posthospital periods have been collected. Prehospital variables include demographic and socioeconomic measures obtained from the patient or from hospital records on admission. In-hospital variables include clinical assessments, treatments provided (excluding medication), behavior changes, and discharge destination. Posthospital variables reflect factors in the patient's life following discharge. The predictor variables are summarized in table 2.1

Patients' progress in hospital treatment, expected to be a key factor, was measured in terms of a system developed for that purpose, the Treatment Progress Scales (TPS; see Schalock, Sheehan & Webster, in press). The conceptual basis for the TPS is that a valid way to measure treatment-related behavior changes is by monitoring the patient's achievement of specific treatment goals developed by the treatment team. This general approach, initially developed by Kiresuk and Sherman (1986) as Goal Attainment Scaling, has been used widely to evaluate client progress and program outcomes in mental

Table 2.1: Management Study Data Sets and Predictor Variables

Prehospital Data[a] *(Collected on admission)*	*In-hospital Data*[b] *(Collected on Discharge)*	*Posthospital Data*[c] *(Collected on Readmission or Followup)*
*1. Age	1. Average TPS change scores	1. Factors contributing to readmission/ non-readmission
*2. Gender	*a. Initial vs 24 hours	*2. Current living environment
*3. Educational level	*b. Initial vs Time 1 (7 days)	*3. Current employment status
*4. Race	*c. Initial vs discharge	*4. Community resources used (sum)
5. Legal status	*d. Time 1 vs discharge	*5. Taking medication on discharge
6. Catchment Area	*2. Allen Cognitive Level	*6. Taking medication as prescribed
*7. Number of previous admissions to HRC	*3. Days of hospitalization	*7. Instrumental activities of daily living (sum)
8. Number of previous admissions to other MH/ alcohol facilities	*4. Hours of individual psychotherapy	*8. Physical health impairments (sum)
*9. Marital status	*5. Hours OT/IT/RT	*9. TPS self-rating
*10. Employment status before	*6. Number of family visits	
	*7. Type of living arrangements following discharge	
	*8. Axis I diagnosis	
	*9. Average TPS self-rating (admission to discharge)	
	10. Changes in adaptive behavior	
	*a. Relationships	
	*b. General physical health	
	*c. Self-image	
	*d. General enjoyment of life	
	*e. Coping skills	

* Denotes a predictor variable in the multiple discriminant analysis.

a. Data sets similar to those used by Goering et al., 1984; Lorei & Gurel, 1973; Rosenblatt & Mayer, 1974; Gribman, Tessler & Wellin, 1987; Lambert et al., 1983; Leff & Vaughn, 1980.

b. Data sets similar to those used by Miller et al., 1984; Vaughn & Leff, 1976. Description of the Treatment Progress Scales (TPS) is found in Schalock, Sheehan & Weber (In press). The Allen Cognitive Level evaluation is described in Allen (1987).

c. Data sets similar to those used by Bland, Parker & Orn (1976); Buell & Anthony (1973); Malone (1989); Mueller (1980); Tessler & Manderschild (1982); Thompson (1985); Turner (1981); Weller & Biggins (1976).

Table 2.2: Treatment Progress Scales (TPS) Problem Areas and Dictionary Examples

PROBLEM AREAS

Activity level	Denial (of problem)	Psychomatic complaints
Agression	Dependency	Sadness or depression
Assertiveness, lack of	Disruptiveness	Secondary adaptation: altered belief or perception
Bizarre habits or rituals	Hallucinations	Self-esteem, lack of
Chemical dependency alcohol other drugs	Judgement, impaired	Self-injury
Coherent speech, lack of	Manipulation	Sexual control, lack of
Compliance, lack of	Memory, lack of	Socialization, lack of
Delusions	Motivation, lack of	Stealing
	Obsessive-compulsive	Suicide
	Obtunded	Suspicion
	Orientation, lack of	
	Psychoactive substance abuse	

TPS DICTIONARY EXAMPLES

Problem Area	*Behavioral Indicator*
Assertiveness, lack of	Number of people spoken to Responds without being prodded Says no Initiates tasks Direct others
Attention, lack of	Follows directions Answers questions Makes eye contact Looks at
Bizarre habits or rituals	Postures with hands and/or feet Filters light through fingers Holds hands in unusual positions Walks forward and then backward when going someplace Steps only on certain tile spaces Ingests objects Eating and/or dressing rituals

health programs, in special education and developmental disability services, and in family therapy.

The TPS includes a standardized list of 34 problem titles, reflecting problems frequently encountered in psychiatric and substance abuse populations (Montgomery et al., 1978). These titles are listed in the top portion of table 2.2

Immediately upon the patient's admission, an individualized problem list is constructed by selecting relevant titles. For each problem, behavioral indicators are selected as descriptors of progress along a 5-point scale: 5 = best anticipated success with treatment; 4 = more than expected success with treatment; 3 = expected level of treatment success; 2 = less than expected success with treatment; 1 = most unfavorable outcome thought likely. Twenty-four hours after admission, a ward nurse evaluates the patient's behavior with respect to progress in each problem area. The treatment team makes subsequent evaluations every seven days in the substance abuse units or every 30 days in the psychiatric units. New progress scales can be developed at any time. A final evaluation is made at discharge.

The quality of each TPS is evaluated according to eight technical standards within seven days of the scale's development. These eight standards, which are applied on a yes/no basis, ask whether the problem behaviors are clearly defined, whether they are measurable, whether they are related to hospital admissions, whether the progress scales are completely defined, whether the scale descriptors are inclusive, whether the descriptors overlap, and whether the descriptors are stated in action verbs.

Following the evaluation under the technical standards, the TPS is entered in a computerized data bank. The data are used to generate TPS reports and graphs on an IBM System /36 using AIMS hospital information system software and SAS statistical software. The graphs are output as PostScript graphics stream files for printing on a PostScript printer. The PostScript graphics stream files are downloaded to a personal computer equipped with JetScript controller card and software from QMS, and are then printed on a Hewlett-Packard LaserJet equipped with a JetScript-adapted card from QMS to make the LaserJet PostScript-compatible. Tables and graphic summaries are available by diagnostic group or by problem area for the individual client, for a ward, or for the total facility.

Table 2.3 summarizes our work to date on three psychometric properties of the TPS, including a brief description of each property and the correspond-

Table 2.3: Treatment Progress Scales (TPS) Psychometric Properties

Property	*Brief Description*	*Psychometric Indices(s)*
1. Normative data	TPS scores and change scores analyzed by diagnostic group and problem area	Scores available on 4600 persons
2. Reliability		
a. Interrate	Consistency between psychiatrist and charge nurse	interrater reliability coefficient $(r) = 0.68$, $df = 398$, $p < .001$
b. Developed within technical standards	Consistency with which treatment goals are developed within 8 technical standards	92 percent of 4600 TPS developed from 1987 to 1991 meet the 8 technical standards
3. Validity		
a. Content	Problem areas included in the TPS are consistent with the content of published psychiatric rating scales (14, 15)	
b. Concurrent	(1) TPS scores vs Brief Psychiatric Rating Scale scores (for comparable problem areas)	(1) Average concurrent validity coefficients = 0.49, $df = 102$, $p < .01$
	(2) TPS scores vs weekly behavioral points[a]	(2) Average concurrent validity coefficients = 0.41, $df = 102$, $p < .01$
c. Construct	Correlation between TPS and other indicators of treatment success	Significant correlations ($df = 398$, $p < .001$) obtained between TPS changes and general physical health ($r = .29$), average ability to cope ($r = .22$), hours in therapeutic activities ($r = .28$), and nonrecidivism ($rps = 0.65$)

Note: See text for explanation of TPS.

a. These points are tabulated daily on a standardized recording sheet by ward personnel. They reflect the patient's involvement in therapeutic programs, completion of personal hygiene and maintenance tasks, following ward and facility policies, and demonstrating prosocial behaviors.

ing psychometric indices. The normative data have been used for comparison purposes and longitudinal program evaluation studies. The two reliability estimates represent the consistency with which clinicians evaluate the behavioral changes and develop treatment goals within accepted technical standards. The three validity coefficients reflect acceptable content and concurrent and construct validity.

Prediction of Rehospitalization

The data were analyzed in a multiple discriminant analysis (MDA) in which the 32 predictor variables were regressed against the dichotomized outcome variables of returned or not returned within the 12-month postdischarge period. MDA is a multivariate technique that distinguishes two or more groups by means of a statistically best combination of variables forming a single profile or function (Nuehring, Thayer & Ladner, 1980). A standardized discriminant coefficient can be used to establish which variables contribute most in distinguishing the groups.

The MDA identified five variables that discriminated significantly between the recidivist and nonrecidivist groups (table 2.4). The canonical discriminant function allowed 85 percent of the cases to be correctly classified.

Note that cognitive level, as measured by the Allen Cognitive Level Test, did not discriminate between recidivists and nonrecidivists. However, as shown in table 2.5, cognitive level correlates positively and significantly with three of the five discriminating variables, including physical and health impairments, educational level, and the initial score on the Treatment Progress Scales vs. the 24-hour score. Table 2.5 also summarizes the significant cor-

Table 2.4: Variables That Discriminate Significantly between Recidivists and Nonrecidivists

Variable	*Characteristic of Recidivists*
Physical/health impairments	Higher number of physical impairments
Previous admission to Hastings Regional Center	More previous admissions
Educational level	Higher educational level
Employment status	Greater likelihood of unemployment
TPS score: Initial vs. 24 hours[a]	Higher TPS score

Note: Based on multiple discriminant analysis; F test significant at .05 or greater level of significance.

a. See text for TPS description.

Table 2.5: Significant Correlations between Assessed Cognitive Level and Demographic Characteristics, Self-sufficiency Measures, and Hospitalization Factors

Demographic Characteristics	*Self-Sufficiency Measures*	*Hospitalization Factors*
Age: –.36**	Employment status: .17**	TPS: initial vs 24 hour: .14*
Gender: .15*	Living arrangement: .31**	TPS: initial vs discharge: .16**
Education level: .27**	Activities of daily living: .40**	Hours of indiv. therapy: .14*
	Health impairments: .18**	Days hospitalized: –.12*

*$p < .05$ ($df = 265$) **$p < .01$ ($df = 265$)

relations between cognitive level and a number of assessed variables, including demographic characteristics, self-sufficiency measures, and hospitalization factors. The implications of these relationships for service planning will be discussed in this chapter's final section.

Cognitive Level and Behavioral Change

The second issue addressed in this chapter is the temporal relationship between measured cognitive changes and assessed behavioral changes. Theoretically, this relationship is relevant to the question of whether cognitive change precedes behavioral change, or vice versa (see chap. 9 of this volume). To evaluate this relationship, the sequential changes in both cognitive level and Treatment Progress Scales were analyzed.

The sequential analysis of cognitive level and behavioral changes was done on a random sample of 40 patients from the Psychiatric Unit at Hastings Regional Center. A purposive random sampling technique was used on patients from four Axis I diagnostic groups: organic personality syndrome, schizophrenia, affective disorders, and adjustment disorders; 10 subjects per group were selected on the basis of a minimum of four sequential cognitive level tests and four sequential measures on one or more Treatment Progress Scales. Characteristics of this sample are summarized in table 2.6, and the sequential cognitive level and TPS data are summarized in table 2.7.

Three general trends are apparent from table 2.7. First, cognitive levels increase sequentially, but, except for the organic personality syndrome diagnosis, they increase only from the first to the second assessment. Thereafter, cognitive level remains quite stable. The trend among schizophrenic patients

Table 2.6: Subject Descriptions Used to Determine Temporal Relationship between Measured Cognitive Changes and Assessed Behavioral Changes

Axis I Diagnosis	*Age*	*Gender*	*Length of Stay (Days)*	*Cognitive Level*[a]
Organic Personality Syndrome	43.4	6 females, 4 males	86.5	3.7 (± 0.6)[b]
Schizophrenia	34.5	5 each	97.3	4.6 (± 0.7)
Affective disorders	45.5	5 each	123.6	4.8 (± 0.9)
Adjustment disorders	29.1	3 females, 7 males	57.3	5.4 (± 0.8)

Note: Data presented are means.

a. Cognitive levels are done upon admission for cognitive training. Repeat levels are done when requested, when change is noticed, or to update information if the length of stay has been extensive.

b. Standard deviation.

is interesting, as the steady decline following the second assessment might reflect the attentional deficit seen frequently in schizophrenic patients. In contrast, TPS scores tend to increase sequentially, to peak at the fifth or sixth assessment.

Implications for Service Planning

A reasonable conclusion from the data summarized in this chapter is that cognitive functioning as assessed by the Allen Cognitive Levels covaries with a number of treatment factors, including TPS changes, hours of therapy received, and number of days of hospitalization. It does not appear that assessed cognitive level is a *predictor variable* for either recidivism or sequential behavioral change. However, assessed cognitive level does correlate significantly with a number of self-sufficiency measures (see table 2.5), some of which are predictive of rehospitalization. In that regard, the data presented also support the construct validity of the Allen Cognitive Level Test in that, as a measure of occupational-functional potential, the test correlates significantly with a number of self-sufficiency measures, including employment status, living arrangement, and level of daily activities. Thus lower cognitive level in a patient should suggest to treatment planners that they pay special

Table 2.7: Sequential Changes in Assessed Cognitive Level and Behavior (TPS)

Axis I Diagnosis	*Cognitive Level Changes*[a]				*TPS Problem Area*	*Behavior TPS Changes*[a]			
	1	2	3	4		1	2	3	4
Organic Personality Disorder	3.9	3.7	3.8	4.0	Verbal hostility	1.6	2.6	4.0	3.8
					Physical aggression	1.8	2.2	3.4	3.6
					Disruptiveness	1.4	1.6	2.2	3.5
Schizophrenia	4.4	4.8	4.6	4.4	Disruptiveness	1.0	2.5	3.0	3.3
					Denial	1.5	2.3	2.3	2.0
					Verbal hostility	1.2	2.4	2.4	4.0
					Delusions	1.1	1.9	2.4	3.0
					Hallucinations	1.0	1.6	2.0	3.0
Affective disorders	4.5	4.9	4.8	4.9	Sadness or depression	1.1	1.5	1.8	3.3
Adjustment disorder	5.1	5.4	5.3	5.6	Sadness or depression	1.1	2.3	2.5	3.8
					Suicide	1.0	2.0	2.5	2.5
Overall mean	4.5	4.7	4.6	4.7		1.2	2.1	2.6	3.3

a. Data presented are mean scores per sequential time period (1–4).

attention to rehabilitation efforts targeting self-sufficiency behaviors such as employment, supportive living arrangements, and activities of daily living.

The finding from the recidivism analysis that the number of reported health impairments was a significant discriminating variable is also consistent with an emerging trend in the psychiatric rehabilitation literature indicating that those hospitalized have more stress-related symptoms and perform fewer activities of daily living (Avison & Speechley, 1987; Goering et al., 1984). Conversely, one finds that a decrease in stress and physical ailments accompanies community stabilization (Wright et al., 1989). Of course, health problems are themselves stressors that may contribute to psychiatric hospitalization.

The fact that those readmitted had also used more community services prior to their rehospitalization is also consistent with previous research (Franklin et al., 1975), and it suggests that such persons are attempting to obtain assistance for their physical and psychiatric symptoms. Thus, such persons may be using the psychiatric hospital as a logical extension of the health care delivery system. This possibility is further augmented by two realities of rural America: first, Medicare and private insurance discriminate against rural services in their reimbursement policies; and second, in rural areas there is a shortage of health personnel (DeLeon et al., 1989), especially those who can deal effectively with chronic patients (Malone, 1989).

The finding of the significant role that physical symptoms and illness play in rehospitalization also suggests that psychiatric facilities would do well to recognize the significant contribution that chronic stress may make to a patient's posthospital course, and the resultant need to focus on the stress-process perspective (Avison & Speechley, 1987) and the person's social support system (Schalock, 1990; Schalock & Kiernan, 1990). Comprehensive stress inoculation and stress management programs initiated in the hospital could better prepare the person for successful posthospital adjustment (Schafer, 1987). The significant negative correlation obtained between health impairments and educational level, and the positive correlation between assessed cognitive level and educational level, suggest that educational programs can be effective in patient-referenced comprehensive stress management programs.

* * *

In summary, assessed cognitive level should play an important part in both planning services and delivering them to psychiatric patients. Although assessed cognitive level may act as an intervening rather than a predictive variable, its demonstrated relationship to self-sufficiency measures and treatment outcome warrants its inclusion in current and future rehabilitative practices.

References

Allen, C. (1986). *Occupational therapy for psychiatric diseases: Measurement and management of cognitive disabilites.* Boston: Little & Brown.

Anthony, W. A., Cohen, M. R., & Vitalo, R. (1978). The measurement of rehabilitation outcome. *Schizophrenia Bulletin,* 4, 375–383.

Avison, W. R., & Speechley, K. N. (1987). The discharged psychiatric patient: A review of social, social-psychological, and psychiatric correlates of outcome. *American Journal of Psychiatry,* 144(1), 10–18.

Bartko, J. J., Carpenter, W. T., & McGlashan, T. H. (1988). Statistical issues in long-term followup studies. *Schizophrenia Bulletin,* 14(4), 575–587.

Bland, R. C., Parker, J. W., & Orn, H. (1976). Prognosis in schizophrenia: A ten year follow-up of first admission. *Archives of General Psychiatry,* 33, 949–954.

Buell, G. J., & Anthony, W. A. (1973). Demographic characteristics as predictors of recidivism and post-hospital employment. *Journal of Counseling Psychology,* 20, 361–365.

DeLeon, P. H., Wakefield, M., Schultz, A. J., Williams, J. & Vanden Box, G. R. (1989). Rural America: Unique opportunities for health care delivery and health services research. *American Psychologist,* 44(10), 1298–1306.

Filskov, S. B., Grimm, G. H., & Lewis, J. A. (1981). Brain-behavior relationships. In S. D. Filskov & T. J. Boll (Eds.), *Handbook of Clinical Neuropsychology,* 147–160. New York: Springer-Verlag.

Franklin, J. L., Kittridge, L. D., & Thrasher, J. H. (1975). A survey of factors related to mental hospital readmissions. *Hospital and Community Psychiatry,* 26(11), 749–751.

Goering, P., Wasylenki, D., Lancee, W., & Freedman, S. J. J. (1984). From hospital to community: Six-month and two-year outcomes for 505 patients. *The Journal of Nervous and Mental Disease,* 172(11), 667–673.

Gribman, G. D., Tessler, R. C., & Wellin, G. (1987). Living with the mentally ill: Factors affecting household complaints. *Schizophrenia Bulletin,* 13(4), 727–736.

Kiresuk, T. J., & Sherman, R. E. (1988). Goal attainment scaling: A general method of evaluation of comprehensive community mental health programs. *Community Mental Health Journal* 4, 443–453.

Lambert, E. W., Sherwood, V., & Fitzpatrick, L. J. (1983). Predicting recidivism among first admissions at Tennessee's state psychiatric hospitals. *Hospital and Community Psychiatry,* 34(10), 951–953.

Leff, J., & Vaughn, C. (1980). The interaction of life events and relatives' expressed emotion in schizophrenia and depressive neurosis. *British Journal of Psychiatry,* 136, 146–153.

Lorei, T. W., & Gurel, L. (1973). Demographic characteristics as predictors of post-hospital employment and readmission. *Journal of Consulting Clinical Psychology,* 40(3), 426–430.

Malone, J. (1989). Concepts for the rehabilitation of the long-term mentally ill in the community. *Issues in Mental Health Nursing,* 10, 121–135.

Miller, D. J., Beck, N. C., & Fraps, C. (1984). Predicting rehospitalization at a community mental health center: A "double crossed" validation. *Journal of Clinical Psychology,* 40(1), 35–39.

Montgomery, L. M., Shadish, W. R., Jr., Orwin, R. G., & Bootzin, R. R. (1978). Psychometric structure of psychiatric rating scales. *Journal of Abnormal Psychology* 96(2), 167–170.

Mueller, D. P. (1980). Social networks: A promising direction for research on the relationship of the social environment to psychiatric disorders. *Social Science Medicine,* 14A, 147–161.

Nuehring, E. M., Thayer, J. H., & Ladner, R. A. (1980). On the factors of predicting rehospitalization among two state mental hospital patient populations. *Administration in Mental Health,* 7(4), 247–270.

Rosenblatt, A., & Mayer, J. E. (1974). The recidivism of mental patients: A review of past studies. *American Journal of Orthopsychiatry,* 44(5), 697–706.

Schafer, W. (1987). *Stress management for wellness.* New York: Holt, Rinehart & Winston.

Schalock, R. L. (1988). *Management study manual.* Hastings, Neb.: Hastings Regional Center.

Schalock, R. L. (1989). *Treatment progress scales: Instruction manual* (2nd edit.). Hastings, Neb.: Hastings Regional Center.

Schalock, R. L. (1990). *Quality of life: Perspectives and issues.* Washington, D.C.: American Association on Mental Retardation.

Schalock, R. L., & Kiernan, W. E. (1990). *Habilitation planning for adults with disabilities.* New York: Springer-Verlag.

Schalock, R. L., Sheehan, M. J., & Weber, L. (In press). The use of treatment progress scales in the client monitoring and evaluation system. *Journal for Mental Health Administration.*

Schalock, R. L., & Thornton, C. V. D. (1988). *Program evaluation: A field guide for administrators.* New York: Plenum Press.

Tessler, R. C., & Manderscheid, R. (1982). Factors affecting adjustment to community living. *Hospital and Community Psychiatry,* 33, 203–207.

Thompson, C. M. (1985). Characteristics associated with outcome in a community mental health partial hospitalization program. *Community Mental Health Journal,* 21(3), 179–188.

Turner, R. J. (1981). Social support as a contingency in psychological well-being. *Journal of Health Science Behavior,* 22, 357–367.

Vaughn, C. E., & Leff, J. R. (1976). The influence of family and social factors on the course of psychiatric illness. *British Journal of Psychiatry,* 129, 125–137.

Weller, R., & Biggins, P. (1976). Comparison of rehospitalized and non-hospitalized psychiatric patients on community adjustment: Self assessment guide. *Psychiatry,* 39, 239–244.

Wright, R. S., Heinman, J. R., Shupe, J., & Olvera, G. (1989). Defining and measuring stabilization of patients during 4 of intensive community support. *American Journal of Psychiatry,* 146(10), 1293–1298.

• 3 •

Neuropsychological Assessment and Consultation in Psychiatric Rehabilitation

Richard C. Erickson

A number of developments during the past decade have generated an increased need for neuropsychological consultation on acute psychiatric wards, particularly for services in Veterans Administration facilities. Since the veteran population is aging, attention to geriatric problems has become a priority in the VA. Also, policies associated with the deinstitutionalization movement, coupled with inadequate community resources, mean that short-stay admissions include the most severely disturbed and impaired chronic patients. They exhibit multiple, severe, life-threatening problems. The typical patient has a history of repeated hospitalizations and of substance abuse and frequently has medical problems associated with aging and poor self-care.

Major psychiatric disorders have come to be understood as species of brain dysfunction (Andreasen, 1984), and neuropsychologists have been pressed into service to help understand the nature of these disorders. Given this biological perspective, psychiatric rehabilitation approaches have emerged that are comparable to rehabilitation approaches for those who have medical and neurological disabilities (Anthony & Liberman, 1986). Initially, these rehabilitation efforts focused on remedying deficits in self-care and social skills and on specifying and supplying community supports needed to maximize chronic patients' functioning in the community (Anthony, 1980; Liberman, 1988). More recently, however, there has been an increasing recognition that these patients suffer from cognitive deficits that undermine their ability to benefit from training programs and to keep up with the demands of community living (Erickson, 1988; Stuve, Erickson & Spaulding, 1991). Such deficiencies are seldom obvious, since few patients appear to be "slow," nor do they perform more poorly on traditional IQ tests than one might expect from their educational and occupational backgrounds.

We thus have reason to hypothesize that a number of chronic patients indeed have significant cognitive deficits related to their primary psychiatric diagnoses, and to the aging process, medical problems, histories of substance abuse, and the like. However, neuropsychologists have not often identified and addressed the functional implications of these deficits. Traditionally, neuropsychologists have seen their role as that of mapping relationships between brain and behavior and of providing answers to differential diagnostic questions about brain-injured patients (Chelune & Moehle, 1986). When confronted with psychiatric patients, neuropsychologists have focused their efforts on searching for markers or patterns associated with various diagnoses or on differentiating between functional and organic causes (Erickson & Binder, 1986; Goldstein, 1978). Recently, however, neuropsychologists have turned their attention from questions of etiology to questions of functional abilities and disabilities and their remediation (Chelune & Moehle, 1986). This perspective initially developed out of experience with brain-injured patients, and the burgeoning field of cognitive rehabilitation is the result (Adamovich et al., 1985; Benedict, 1989; Christensen & Uzell, 1988; Diller & Gordon, 1981a, 1981b; Edelstein & Coulture, 1984; Goldstein & Ruthven, 1983; Gouvier et al., 1986; Grimm & Bleiberg, 1986; Gummow et al., 1983; Meier et al., 1987; Prigatano, 1986; Sohlberg & Mateer, 1989; Trexler, 1982; Wilson, 1987). More recently, this functional perspective has been applied to the cognitive assessment and remediation of deficits experienced by persons with severe and persistent psychiatric conditions (Diamant, 1981, 1985; Diamant & Huijsman, 1982; Erickson, 1988; Erickson & Binder, 1986; Erickson & Burton, 1986; Spaulding et al., 1986; Stuve, Erickson & Spaulding, 1991; Townes et al., 1985; Yozawitz, 1986).

This chapter first describes a consultative approach to psychiatric patients developed at the Portland, Oregon and Brockton–West Roxbury, Massachusetts VA medical centers in collaboration with occupational therapists at the two facilities. The chapter then makes some preliminary observations about the state of the art and the tasks that lie ahead.

A Consultative Approach

The development of the test protocol used in the consultative approach has been discussed in previous publications (Erickson & Binder, 1986; Erickson,

1988), so the process will be only briefly outlined here. The first step was awareness that chronic psychiatric patients have subtle but significant cognitive deficits that hamper their ability to benefit from treatment and to function in the community. The second step involved a shift from asking diagnostic questions to asking questions about functional abilities and disabilities. This step was reinforced by the work by Townes et al. (1985) demonstrating a lack of correlation between diagnoses and patterns of cognitive deficits, as well as collaborative relationships between this author and occupational therapists. The third step identified tests of higher neuropsychological functioning that appeared to be analogous to tasks of daily living (Erickson & Binder, 1986), and, at the same time, identified psychosocial interventions that could plausibly be regarded as relevant for addressing the deficits found (Erickson & Burton, 1986; Erickson, 1989).

This approach has been constrained by the settings in which it is to be applied: short-stay admitting wards where acutely disturbed patients are treated and discharged in a matter of a few weeks. Under such circumstances, assessment cannot properly be undertaken until the acute symptomatology is brought under control and patients reach the point of being "as good as they are going to get." Consequently, testing takes place relatively late in the hospital stay of most patients, leaving precious little time to undertake sustained rehabilitation efforts. The result is an emphasis on the role of consultant: reporting findings and making recommendations to patients and their families, to staff, and to community caregivers.

ILLUSTRATIVE DATA

The inpatient unit at Portland VA Medical Center is a typical short-stay psychiatric unit in the VA system serving adult patients with a wide range of chronic psychiatric disorders. On this unit a testing protocol was developed that contrasted "old learning" (as measured by education and vocabulary from our routinely given Self Administered Battery [Lezak, 1983]) and current adaptive abilities. The protocol includes tests of attention and concentration, learning and memory, psychomotor speed, and problem solving (Erickson & Binder, 1986). The protocol, which takes about an hour to administer, includes Digit Span, the Inglis Paired Associates, Babcock Story Recall, Digit Symbol, Trails B, Block Design, Rey Complex Figure Test (CFT), Wisconsin Card Sort Test, and WAIS Comprehension. This contrasting of old learning and current adaptive abilities is echoed in Sternberg's automatized vs. nonintrenched tasks, Horn's crystallized vs. fluid abilities, and Schneider and Shiffren's automatic vs. controlled or effortful information processing. Current adaptive abilities appear to be more vulnerable to age and pathology than is the case with old learning. Depending on the patient's performance, other tasks may be added to tease out further information or to test specific hypotheses.

A sample of 100 completed protocols for 50 schizophrenic and 50 nonschizophrenic patients randomly drawn from the test files of the Portland inpatient unit serves to illustrate key points. The data in the files had not been randomly obtained from all admissions to the ward. Patients had been selected for testing for a variety of reasons, including histories of substance abuse, vague or unusual medical histories that would not lend themselves to the formulation of a clear-cut neuropsychological referral question, or disappointing responses to treatment interventions. The patients were tested when they were judged to be "as good as they were going to get" in the hospital. In the case of alcoholic patients, there was an interval of at least 7–10 days postadmission, and in the case of other patients, testing waited until they became medically and psychiatrically stable. Given problems of treatment compliance and the relative inadequacy of community supports and follow-up options, it can be argued that testing was administered at a time when most of these patients were functioning at their best.

Table 3.1 shows the number of patients who scored at or below a cutoff point indicating below-average or impaired performance for the test in question. The cutoff points chosen included Education < 10th grade, SABT Vocabulary < 13, WAIS Digit Span < 8, Inglis Paired Associates > 10, Story Recall < 12, Trails B < 25th percentile (age corrected), Rey CFT approach fragmented and disorganized (Lezak, 1983), WAIS-R Block Design SS < (8), WAIS-R Comprehension SS < (8), Wisconsin Card Sort < 3 categories in 128 trials or > 40 trials without attaining a category. (Refer to the WAIS-R manual, Inglis's [1959], or Lezak's [1983] text for particulars about the tests and their scoring.)

The sample of 100 patients had a median age of 40 years ($R = 23-74$) and a median education of 12 years ($R = 7-16+$). Sixty-one of the patients had documented problems with substance abuse, about equally distributed between the two groups.

Inspection of the data in table 3.1 suggests several things. First, old learn-

Table 3.1: Number of Subjects Showing Impaired Performance

	Old learning		*Information Processing*				*Psychomotor Speed*			*Problem Solving*			
Group	*Educ.*	*Vocab.*	*Digit Span*	*Inglis*	*Story Recall*	*Story Del.*	*Digit Symbol*	*Trails B*	*Rey CFT*	*Block Design*	*WAIS Comp.*	*Wisc. CST*	*Mean*
Schiz. ($n = 50$)	9	6	12	28	26	35	42	34	34	26	19	34	30.89
Nonschiz. ($n = 50$)	9	8	9	28	29	28	34	23	24	19	13	26	24.89
Total	18	14	21	56	55	63	76	57	58	45	32	60	55.78

ing as measured by education and vocabulary ($Md = 19.5, R = 6–25$) appears no more frequently below average than one might expect from a general or veteran population. Similarly, impairment on Digit Span appears no more frequently than expected. On the other hand, deficiencies in current information processing and memory, psychomotor speed, and problem solving appear characteristic of these patients, with half or more scoring poorly on most of these tasks.

While group comparisons were not the purpose of testing, several results bear consideration in this regard (see table 3.2). First, a comparison of the number of the nine tests failed by the same subject suggests some tendency for patients who fail some tests of current adaptive abilities to fail many, and a tendency for schizophrenic patients to fail pervasively more than non-schizophrenic patients (chi-square = 5.25 1 *df*, $p < .05$; see table 3.2a). Patients with the lowest vocabulary scores do more poorly than patients with the highest (chi-square = 3.57 1 *df*, $p < .06$, see table 3.2b). There is no significant tendency for patients with substance abuse problems to fail more tests than those who are not substance abusers (chi-square < 1 1 *df*; see table 3.2c). None of this is particularly surprising, but as the categorical data suggest, neither are the effects very striking, except in the case of patients with below-average levels of intellectual functioning as measured by vocabulary.

The data presented here support the arguments of Townes et al. (1985), Erickson (1988), Erickson and Binder (1986), Spaulding et al. (1986), and Yozawitz (1986). Cognitive assessments of psychiatric patients do more than repeat information that could be inferred from IQ or diagnosis. Though it is true that some patients who tend to do poorly on some of the tests of current adaptive abilities also tend to do poorly on others, for rehabilitation purposes it seems wise to ascertain the profile of cognitive strengths and weaknesses peculiar to each individual.

CONSULTATIVE INTERVENTIONS

The assessment contributes in several ways to the rehabilitation of the patient (Erickson & Burton, 1986). First, it informs clinical decisions about suitable placements: Should the patient continue to live independently, or should he or she be directed to a supervised living situation such as a family home, a foster home, a nursing home, or even an open or locked chronic care ward in a hospital facility? Second, it forms the basis for recommendations to hospital

Table 3.2: Number of Patients Failing Multiple Tests

Number of tests failed	A. Diagnosis		B. Vocabulary		C. Substance abuse	
	Schiz.	Nonschiz.	< 13	> 13	Yes	No
0–4	12	24	5	10	22	14
5–9	38	26	21	10	39	25

and community caregivers about how best to understand and approach the problems presented by the patient. Caregivers often express vague or misguided concerns. They are aware that the patient is not functioning as expected, but they may attribute such failure to a direct effect of the illness, to some vaguely described cognitive deficit ("poor memory"), or to lack of motivation or lack of cooperation (describing the patient as "manipulative," "treatment-resistant," "passive/aggressive," and the like). Such misattributions often lead to inappropriate and counterproductive expectations and emotional responses. Clarification of the specific nature of the patient's cognitive deficits can result in more appropriate individual and group interventions (Erickson, 1989) instead of exasperation and mutual recrimination. Finally, a patient may benefit from being told about the specific nature of his or her deficits and about how to correct the problems or how to employ "prosthetic devices" to work around the problems. Assessment may suggest systematic training programs that can teach needed cognitive skills, substitute skills, or the skills needed to employ prosthetic devices effectively (Stuve, Erickson & Spaulding, 1991). Though such systematic training programs are often beyond the capabilities of consultants associated with acute psychiatric units, the assessments can form the basis for appropriate referrals or follow-up activities.

The State of the Art

It is evident that we are engaged in developing a new clinical specialty or subspecialty: assessing and remediating cognitive deficits among chronic psychiatric patients. We work in facilities serving psychiatric patients, and this focus sets us apart from colleagues who are working with head-injured patients. Within psychiatric settings, we claim to possess expertise that fellow clinicians do not have. Our status as experts in this emerging field requires that we be fully aware of the state of the art and of the work that still needs to be done. As we strive to establish our identity, and the credibility of our work both as individuals and as a group of specialists, several interrelated questions arise.

1. *How is the present enterprise related to the parent disciplines?*

We come to our present situations from differing educational and experiential backgrounds. We are indebted to existing specialties and disciplines for many of the conceptual and practical tools that we employ, for professional access to the clinical populations we serve, and for ensuring that our contributions will be received as credible by other disciplines and by patients and their families. At the same time, we are attempting to develop distinct new perspectives, concepts, and practices. This point can be clearly illustrated with reference to psychology. Within the broader field of clinical psychology, we do not present ourselves as uniquely skilled in making psychiatric diagnoses or in conducting "psychotherapy." Rather we define ourselves as knowledgeable in the assessment and treatment of functional cognitive abilities and deficits. More than a shift of emphasis is involved in this redefinition. As we noted earlier, patterns of cognitive abilities and deficits relate poorly to psychiatric diagnoses, and the kinds of questions we ask differ from those traditionally asked by clinical psychologists. In the parent discipline, treatment follows from and is informed by Axis I and Axis II diagnoses; in our venture, clinical efforts presuppose the existence of some severe and persistent psychiatric condition, but they require distinct assessment procedures and interpretive principles as well as distinct remedial efforts.

Similarly, we are indebted to the fields of neuropsychology and cognitive rehabilitation for many of the conceptual and practical tools we employ. At the present time, we properly borrow in wholesale fashion, but it is unlikely that this procedure will continue indefinitely. For one reason, we are not interested in assessing or treating a wide range of basic speech, language, and visuo-spatial deficits. For another, as we come to understand better the nature of cognitive dysfunction in psychiatric populations and as we develop more numerous and refined techniques for addressing various kinds of cognitive deficits, the populations we serve will likely require differing foci of attention.

Additionally, we are already part of and indebted to a broader rehabilitation enterprise. As a group, rehabilitation professionals presuppose the establishment of a medical or psychiatric diagnosis and the implementation of appropriate medical or psychiatric interventions. The rehabilitation professional regards the patient as medically or psychiatrically "stable"; the task of rehabilitation is to address existing functional deficits using physical, psychological, and/or socio-environmental interventions. However, the traditional focus of rehabilitation psychologists has been helping patients to achieve various educational or vocational goals and, more recently, helping them achieve better instrumental and social skills. The present enterprise focuses on underlying cognitive skills and deficits.

Finally, the present enterprise is informed by the cognitive sciences in general and by cognitive psychology and the study of intelligence in particular. Since this point is less obvious, I would like to discuss it at some length. The preoccupations of many cognitive psychologists seem far removed from clinical problems. Nevertheless, they indeed offer something that clinicians need: systematic analyses of the processes of learning and memory, problem solving, and the like, as well as comprehensive, systematic, and articulate theoretical schemes for approaching clinical problems in a better-organized and more focused fashion.

Most would agree that cognitive psychology enjoys no theoretical consensus at the present time. However, the work of Robert Sternberg and his colleagues (Sternberg 1985, 1988, 1990; Sternberg & Smith, 1986; Sternberg & Wagner, 1987) provides a particularly promising new way of approaching the question of "intelligence." First, Sternberg (1990) has written a well-organized and readable account of historical and contemporary theories of intelligence subsumed under seven "metaphors": geographical, computational, biological, epistomological, anthropological, sociological, and systems-oriented. His timely overview can acquaint readers with the wide variety of ways of thinking about intelligent behavior, including concepts used and how they are measured, as well as helping readers to see various theories in relationship to one another.

One collection of papers systematically discusses various aspects of human thought—e.g., induction, deduction, judgment and decision making, problem solving, etc. (Sternberg and Smith, 1986). Another collection examines the study of practical intelligence, i.e., intelligence operating in the everyday world, as opposed to academic settings (Sternberg and Wagner, 1989). This emphasis is important because intelligence and intelligence testing have traditionally been associated with and validated on academic performance. Sternberg's contribution is broadening the definition of intelligence to include the "purposive adaptation, and selection and shaping of real world environments relevant to one's life" (Sternberg, 1985, p.45). Despite this advance, however, his notion of practical intelligence has not been worked out for the chronic patient populations that concern us.

Finally, Sternberg presents a comprehensive triarchic theory of human intelligence in both technical (1985) and popular writing (1988). Space will not permit an elaboration of this theory, so the reader is referred to the books themsleves for a more thorough discussion (particularly to pp. 320–21 in his 1985 book for a presentation of the components of the theory and their relationships). His is a systems theory comprised of a componential subtheory including fluid and crystallized abilities, an experiential subtheory about the abilities to deal with novelty and to automatize information processing, and a contextual subtheory having to do with practical and social intelligence. The componential subtheory relates intelligence to the individual's internal world and specifies a set of mental mechanisms that underlie intelligent behavior. The experiential subtheory relates intelligence to both internal and external worlds, relating the exhibition of intelligence in a given task or situation to the amount of experience with the task or situation. The contextual subtheory relates intelligence to the external world, addressing questions of what behaviors are considered intelligent and where they are seen as such.

I have included this brief overview of Sternberg's theory because even within the vast and sometimes impenetrable world of cognitive psychology and the study of intelligence, at least one comprehensive, systematic, and well-articulated theory of intelligent behavior touches upon, albeit in a general way, issues that concern us. It can provide a starting point for developing a comprehensive theoretical structure to guide our efforts in cognitive rehabilitation.

2. *How will we map the emerging domain and what tools will we employ to do our work?*

We have anticipated part of the answer to this question in the process of answering the previous one. We are not primarily engaged in identifying markers or patterns associated with various psychiatric diagnoses, nor are we primarily concerned with relating test behavior to brain dysfunction as such. We are interested instead in relating test behaviors to everyday behaviors, i.e., we are attempting to map and measure intelligent behavior as it relates to living, learning, and working environments (Anthony, 1980). Moreover, given the nature of the chronically impaired population we work with, we are not primarily concerned with answering academic or vocational questions. Rather, we are interested in specific test behaviors as they relate to specific everyday behaviors in the home and in the community.

The first set of issues we encounter has to do with the kind of environments where the patient is expected to function. What specific environmental demands does the patient face? How much support and structure are available in the environments the patient will inhabit? Clinicians usually have little specific information about the environments the patient will live in or about the availability and skills of supportive others, so more systematic ways of assessing these situations need to be developed.

Second, we need to assess the patient's existing repertoire of overlearned behaviors. We usually rely on the patient's educational and occupational achievements or some measure of general level of intellectual functioning, like IQ or vocabulary, to give us a general estimate of the patient' premorbid abilities. This estimate can be compared with various measures of current adaptive abilities to help identify specific cognitive deficits. However, none of these measures directly tells us what specific everyday skills will be found to be overlearned. For example, a housewife confronted with the need to prepare a meal can rely on overlearned skills; a widowed male may find the same task complex and challenging.

Third, we need to select a finite set of tests that will assess the patient's ability to adapt to novel and complex environmental demands. An ideal protocol would assess attention and concentration, learning and memory, psychomotor speed and problem-solving abilities. These tests provide behavioral analogs that could shed light on the tasks of daily living. The length of the protocol should be limited so that it can be employed in a clinical setting.

There are a number of general principles of psychological assessment that guide test protocol development. First, no single test can be expected to serve as an all-purpose tool for assessing all of the relevant cognitive variables. Single instruments such as the Rey Complex Figure Test, the Wisconsin Card Sort Test, and the Allen Cognitive Level Test are all rich and suggestive in terms of the information they provide about current adaptive abilities, but they are limited in the number of cognitive operations they highlight. Second, traditional measures of intellectual functioning (e.g., the WAIS-R) and neuropsychological batteries (e.g., the Halstead-Reitan or Luria-Nebraska neuropsychological battery) were not originally designed for rehabilitation purposes. They lack measures of cognitive skills of interest and include tasks that do not commend themselves as behavioral analogs.

Data from a well-selected set of specific tests may be more useful. For example, work in cognitive psychology and neuropsychology has shown the need to discriminate between measures in terms of attention and concentration, learning and memory, and problem solving. Within such categories, further distinctions are important: verbal and nonverbal memory, and immediate vs. delayed recall. Most recently, an important distinction has been made between declarative and procedural memory (Cohen & Squires, 1980): some patients who do poorly on traditional (declarative) measures show improvement on tasks they have practiced (procedural) even when they cannot recall having done them before.

I have emphasized the need for selecting tests that function as behavioral analogs: tests that will measure level of performance on cognitive variables of interest and that will in some way mirror cognition in action in everyday life. More specifically, we want to select tests that will enable us to see in clinically useful ways how a patient goes about succeeding or failing. This so-called "process approach" (Kaplan, 1988; Lezak, 1983; Luria, 1966, 1973) can supply valuable clues for intervention: ways to teach the patient to approach the cognitive task differently and more effectively.

The number of concepts and tasks we could employ could multiply indefinitely, as one can see by surveying the cognitive and neuropsychological literatures. We can assume, however, that not all distictions are clinically significant for our purposes and that many tasks will prove to be functionally equivalent and thus redundant from a rehabilitation point of view.

3. *How will we establish a common language?*

Some of the language that clinicians employ is borrowed from everyday discourse and can thus conceal a variety of meanings. Some is borrowed from parent disciplines, so the meaning is not always clear to outsiders. Sometimes the way concepts are used varies from discipline to discipline and from practitioner to practitioner.

The need to establish a common language is as important as the task is difficult. One temptation is to create an arcane new language that permits practitioners to communicate with one another with efficiency and precision and that serves to protect guild prerogatives. However, this also hampers communication with other disciplines and with patients and their families. A better alternative would be to establish a comprehensive and agreed-upon cognitive taxonomy using everyday language. Care should be taken to define terms precisely enought so that practitioners can communicate efficiently while, at

Table 3.3: Proposed Cognitive Taxonomy for Rehabilitation

I. Contextual considerations
   A. Type of environment patient must adapt to (living, learning, working)
   B. Difficulty of environmental demands (simple/complex, familiar/novel, time pressures)
   C. Behavioral repertoire (automatized or habitual vs capacity to respond to novelty)
   D. Amount of structure provided by the examiner, environment, test
   E. Goal of clinical involvement (teach patient to adapt to or shape present environment vs change to a more fitting environment)

II. Cognitive capacities and operations
   A. Attention and concentration
      1. Adequate attention span (Digit Span)
      2. Ability to focus on relevant information
      3. Ability to maintain focus in the face of distractors (Stroop Color-Word Test)
      4. Ability to manipulate symbols and icons in working memory (Digits Backward, serial arithmetic)
      5. Ability to shift focus of attention among competing stimuli (Trails B)
      6. Ability to respond simultaneously to multiple tasks (divided attention)
   B. Ability to learn and remember
      1. Type of memory system involved
         a. Verbal vs nonverbal memory
         b. Declarative (facts and ideas) vs procedural (strategies) memory
         c. Type of materials involved (list, paired associate, narrative, etc.)
      2. Acquisition of new information
         a. Ability to comprehend simple and complex information
         b. Ability to organize and rehearse new information and relate it to existing information
      3. Retrieval of learned information
         a. Immediate vs delayed recall
         b. Amount of cuing required (free vs cued recall vs multiple choice recognition
         c. Errors of omission/commission
   C. Ability to respond rapidly to simple, complex, competing stimuli (Trails A & B, Digit Symbol)
   D. Ability to use information to solve problems
      1. Ability to recognize that a problem exists

Table 3.3: Proposed Cognitive Taxonomy for Rehabilitation (*cont.*)

2. Ability to define or redefine a problem so that it can be addressed
3. Ability to establish overall or long-term goals and/or specific or short-term goals
4. Ability to generate multiple solutions to a problem (verbal fluency)
5. Ability to use reasoning processes to organize a response
   a. Ability to discover relationships between objects or events (part/whole, similarities, differences)
   b. Ability to differentiate important and/or central features from trivial details
   c. Ability to use analytic (whole to part) and synthetic (part to whole) reasoning processes (Block Designs, Rey Complex Figure, Hooper VOT)
   d. Ability to use inductive (specific to general) reasoning (series completions, analogies, classification)
   e. Ability to use deductive (general to specific) reasoning (math and logic problems)
   f. Ability to think abstractly (similarities, proverbs)
   g. Ability to plan an orderly sequence of steps that will lead to a solution to the problem (vs trial and error)
   h. Ability to anticipate consequences (cause and effect, necessary and sufficient conditions)
6. Ability to execute plans efficiently and effectively
   a. Ability to delay a response until sufficient thinking and planning has taken place (impulsive vs reflective vs obsessive style)
   b. Ability to make a decision and initiate action
   c. Ability to follow an orderly plan over time
   d. Ability to allocate time wisely
   e. Ability to monitor progress toward the goal (vs doing and undoing)
   f. Ability to persevere in the face of frustration
   g. Ability to evaluate the appropriateness of the response (judgment, quality control, error monitoring)
   h. Ability to change approach on the basis of new information (flexibility vs rigidity-perseveration, Wisconsin Card Sort Test)
7. Ability to generalize knowledge and skills to new situations.

Note: The author is indebted for the concepts and organization in table 3.3 to the work of Sternberg and Mateer.

the same time, keeping the terms close enough to everyday language so that allied professionals and laypersons can understand them. In rehabilitation, our goal is not so much to do things to others as to enlist others to work with us to accomplish goals. We can do this only if we present our findings and recommendations in understandable language.

A functional cognitive language and classification system for rehabilitation is outlined in table 3.3. Exemplary tests and exploratory phrases (in parentheses) are included to further clarify the meaning of some of the items. The cognitive operations listed are not mutually exclusive. There is some overlap and some items are more inclusive than others, e.g., analytic and synthetic reasoning processes. In the assessment literature, there is not to be found a comprehensive listing that neatly arranges all relevant concepts in mutually exclusive or hierarchical ways. Some of the cognitive operations listed in table 3.3 can be directly assessed by means of clinical instruments. Others must be inferred from analysis of a patient's behaviors on a given task or from observations of his or her behavior over the course of the examination.

4. *How will performance in the testing situation relate to the demands of everyday living?*

The parent disciplines have, by and large, avoided answering this question. Tests have been validated by demonstrating their relationship to academic performance, their relationships with other tests purporting to measure the same construct, or their ability to discriminate among known diagnostic groups (see Lezak, 1983; Willis & Schaie, 1986). Demonstrated relationships between test performance and performance in everyday life (apart from academic performance) are generally absent, nonspecific, or minimal (Baddeley et al., 1982; Chelune & Moehle, 1986; Erickson & Binder, 1986; Erickson et al., 1980; Heaton & Pendleton, 1981). The very nature of our enterprise, however, requires us to demonstrate that our assessment tools reflect and predict everyday behavior.

It is impossible to replicate every conceivable circumstance of everyday life during our assessment. Of necessity, we must focus on a finite number of critical behaviors or relevant cognitive operations and represent them in paradigmatic form. Three strategies are commonly employed: simulation, trait or behavioral checklists, and psychometric testing (Sternberg, 1985).

A. *Simulation.* Patients are asked to demonstrate their ability to carry out important functions like cooking a meal, taking medication, making change, balancing a checkbook, or driving a car. Occupational therapists have taken the lead in doing this kind of assessment and there is at least one protocol, the Kohlman Evaluation of Living Skills (Kohlman-McGourty, 1979), that uses this approach to assess a variety of everyday behaviors. Sternberg (1985) also makes reference to the ETS Basic Skills Test, a 65-item measure designed to assess real-life competencies. Two questions arise with this approach. First, do the skills chosen represent an adequate sampling of the everyday behaviors needed to function independently in the community? Second, will behaviors exhibited in a highly structured testing situation be replicated in less structured situations requiring self-initiated behaviors?

B. *Checklists.* Patients may be asked to give self-reports of their experiences, or caregivers may be asked to report on their observations of the patient. Of the many checklists in the psychological and psychiatric literature, most focus on symptomatology and/or personal or social skills rather than cognitive skills. Though several checklist measures of memory abilities are used with the aged (in Poon et al., 1986), none broadly assesses cognitive operations and related everyday activities. Table 3.4 lists items from a checklist developed at the Brockton VAMC. Patients are asked to respond on the basis of their experience to each item, using a five-point rating scale (from "never" to "always"), and caregivers are asked to respond on the basis of their observations and/or on the basis of their experienced need to assist the patient.

Information from such checklists can be quite helpful. Patients and their families are seldom equipped to describe the problems facing them in precise or clinically useful ways. In answering questionnaires they can describe specifically and accurately what needs should be addressed. Clinicians can use the checklist to encourage the respondents to reflect on the full range of behaviors in question. But such instruments have their limits. Self-reports may not accurately reflect everyday functioning, and the reports of patients, families, and test findings are often poorly correlated.

C. *Psychometric Testing.* This involves tasks that purport to measure cognitive operations of interest. Such a reductionistic approach does have advantages in that it highlights and operationalizes the concepts used, quantifies the data, and permits us to answer certain questions about the reliability and validity of

Table 3.4: Cognitive Skills Checklist

Attention and Concentration

___ lost track of date and time
___ seemed confused, wandered off, or got lost
___ followed a daily routine independently
___ understood what he/she heard or read
___ was able to clearly express him/herself
___ had to have things explained to him/her
___ followed directions
___ seemed absentminded
___ seemed to get distracted in the middle of things
___ lost track of what he/she was doing or talking about
___ had trouble following a conversation
___ just stared into space
___ had trouble concentrating

Remembering Things

___ remembered birthdays, holidays, anniversaries, etc.
___ remembered where he/she left things
___ had to be reminded what to do
___ forgot to keep appointments, go to social events, etc.
___ forgot to take medication
___ seemed to pick up new information readily (people's names, current events, etc.)
___ asked the same questions over and over
___ remembered familiar people's names

Solving Problems

___ seemed mentally "slower" than others
___ started activities on his/her own
___ made the same mistakes over and over
___ seemed confused by changes in routine
___ finished what he/she started
___ slept or sat around unless told to do something
___ showed common sense
___ did things that seemed foolish or dangerous
___ had (made) reasonable plans and ideas
___ carried out activities in an orderly way
___ did things impulsively
___ adapted to unexpected events

Table 3.4: Cognitive Skills Checklist (*cont.*)

___ made good decisions
___ planned ahead
___ got stuck on particular ways of thinking or doing things (rigid)
___ solved practical problems
___ recognized and corrected his/her own mistakes
___ considered several possibilities before settling on a preferred course of action
___ appropriately asked for help when needed

Getting Around

___ kept him/herself clean (bathed, washed hair, etc.) brushed teeth, shaved, combed hair
___ planned and cooked his/her own meals
___ ate a proper diet
___ showed good table manners
___ got to places on his/her own (transportation)
___ spent his/her own money wisely
___ did his/her own shopping for food and personal items
___ independently did routine tasks around the house (picked up, cleaned house, washed dishes, did laundry, home repairs, etc.)
___ planned and carried out his/her own activities
___ seemed tactless, insensitive, or intolerant of others

---

the tests used. The disadvantage is a serious question about the "ecological validity" of many of the tasks. As much as possible, tasks should be behaviorally analogous to everyday tasks. However, "there would seem to be a substantial gap between the kinds of real-world adaptation required for everyday functioning and the kinds of adaptation required for performing testlike and laboratory tasks" (Sternberg, 1985, p.29). Furthermore, correlations among tests purporting to measure similar operations are frequently disappointing, and validation of these tests in everyday behavior is rare (Erickson & Binder, 1986; Heaton, Chelune & Lehman, 1978; Heaton & Pendleton, 1981).

* * *

In summary, the need to relate the behaviors we assess and observe in the clinical setting to behaviors exhibited in everyday life in the community is a critical one for our clinical enterprise. We cannot take refuge in diagnostic categories or hypothetical constructs: our claims of expertise rest on the assumption that our assessments will accurately reflect and predict everyday functioning. To date, we have little data to support these claims. However, based on clinical experience and limited systematic experimentation, there is reason to believe that further research will show neuropsychological assessment and consultation to be a valuable component of psychiatric rehabilitation. On the other hand, one can also expect that further research will demonstrate that many of our cherished assumptions are faulty and that some of what we do is both inefficient and ineffective. There is no lack of work to do.

References

Adamovich, B. B., Henderson, J. A., & Auerbach, S. (1985). *Cognitive rehabilitation of closed-head-injured patients: A dynamic approach.* San Diego: College-Hill.

Andreasen, N. C. (1984). *The broken brain.* New York: Harper and Row.

Anthony, W. A. (1980). *The principles of psychiatric rehabilitation.* Baltimore, Md.: University Park Press.

Anthony, W. A., & Liberman, R. P. (1986). The practice of psychiatric rehabilitation: Historical, conceptual, and research base. *Schizophrenic Bulletin,* 12, 542–559.

Baddeley, A., Sunderland, A., & Harris, J. (1982). How well do laboratory-based psychological tests predict patients' performance outside the laboratory? In S. Corkin et al. (Eds.), *Alzheimer's disease: A report of progress.* New York: Raven.

Benedict, R. H. B. (1989). The effectiveness of cognitive remediation strategies for victims of traumatic head-injury: A review of the literature. *Clinical Psychology Review,* 9, 605–626.

Chelune, G. J., & Moehle, K. A. (1986). Neuropsychological assessment and everyday functioning. In D. Wedding, A. M. Horton, & J. Webster (Eds.), *The neuropsychology handbook* (pp. 489–525). New York: Springer Publishing Co.

Christensen, A. L., & Uzell, P. B. (1988). *Neuropsychological rehabilitation.* Boston: Kluwer.

Cohen, N. J., & Squires, L. R. (1980). Preserved learning and retention of pattern analyzing skill in amnesics: Dissociation of knowing how and knowing that. *Science,* 210, 207–209.

Diamant, J. J. (1981, February). Neuropsychological assessment and rehabilitation of patients with psychiatric disorders. In A. Yozawitz (Chair), Cerebral dysfunctions and psychiatric disorders. Symposium conducted at the meeting of the International Neuropsychological Society, Atlanta, Ga.

Diamant, J. J. (1985, April). Specific features of cognitive rehabilitation of psychiatric patients. Paper presented at the Fifth International Symposium, Models and Techniques of Cognitive Rehabilitation, Indianapolis, Ind.

Diamant, J. J., & Huijsman, A. M. (1982). Neuropsychological rehabilitation of psychiatric patients with brain dysfunction: A case study. *Clinical Neuropsychology,* 4, 1–4.

Diller, L., & Gordon, W. A. (1981a). Interventions for cognitive deficits in brain-injured adults. *Journal of Consulting and Clinical Psychology,* 49, 822–834.

Diller, L., & Gordon, W. A. (1981b). Rehabilitation and clinical neuropsychology. In S. B. Filskov & T. J. Boll (Eds.), *Handbook of clinical neuropsychology* (pp. 702–733). New York: Wiley.

Edelstein, B. A., & Coulture, E. T. (Eds.) (1984). *Behavioral assessment and rehabilitation of the traumatically brain injured.* New York: Plenum.

Erickson, R. C. (1988). Neuropsychological assessment and the rehabilitation of persons with severe psychiatric disabilities. *Rehabilitation Psychology,* 33, 15–25.

Erickson, R. C. (1989). Applications of cognitive testing to group therapies with the chronically mentally ill. *International Journal of Group Psychotherapy,* 39, 223–235.

Erickson, R. C., & Binder, L. M. (1986). Cognitive deficits among functionally psychotic patients: A rehabilitation perspective. *Journal of Clinical and Experimental Neuropsychology,* 8, 257–274.

Erickson, R. C., & Burton, M. A. (1986). Working with psychiatric patients with cognitive deficits. *Cognitive Rehabilitation,* 4(4), 26–31.

Erickson, R. C., Poon, L. W., & Walsh-Sweeney, L. (1980). Clinical memory testing of the elderly. In L. W. Poon, J. L. Fozard, L. S. Cermak, D. Arenberg, & L. W. Thompson (Eds.), *New directions in memory and aging* (pp. 379–402). Hillsdale, N. J.: Erlbaum.

Goldstein, G. (1978). Cognitive and perceptual differences between schizophrenics and organics. *Schizophrenia Bulletin,* 4, 160–185.

Goldstein, G., & Ruthven, L. (1983). *Rehabilitation of the brain-injured adult.* New York: Plenum.

Gouvier, D., Webster, J. S., & Blanton, P. D. (1986). Cognitive retraining with brain-damaged patients. In D. Wedding, A. M. Horton, Jr., & J. Webster (Eds.), *The neuropsychology handbook: Behavioral and clinical perspectives* (pp. 278–324). New York: Springer.

Grimm, B. H., & Bleiberg, J. (1986). Psychological rehabilitation in traumatic brain injury. In S. B. Filskov & T. J. Boll (Eds.), *Handbook of clinical neuropsychology,* Vol. 2 (pp. 495–560). New York: Wiley.

Gummow, L., Miller, P., & Dustman, R. E. (1983). Attention and brain injury: A case for cognitive rehabilitation of attentional deficits. *Clinical Psychology Review,* 3, 255–274.

Heaton, R. K., Chelune, G. J., & Lehman, R. A. W. (1978). Using neuropsychological and personality tests to assess the likelihood of patient employment. *Journal of Nervous and Mental Disease,* 166, 408–416.

Heaton, R. K., & Pendleton, M. G. (1981). Use of neuropsychological tests to predict adult patients' everyday functioning. *Journal of Clinical and Consulting Psychology*, 49, 807–821.

Inglis, J. (1959). Learning, retention and conceptual usage in elderly patients with memory disorders. *Journal of Abnormal and Social Psychology*, 51, 210–215.

Kaplan, E. (1988). A process approach to neuropsychological assessment. In T. Boll & B. K. Bryant (Eds.), *Clinical Neuropsychology and Brain Function: Research, Measurement and Practice* (pp. 129–167). Washington, D.C.: American Psychological Association.

Kohlman-McGourty, L. (1979). *Kohlman Evaluation of Living Skills*. Seattle: Author.

Lezak, M. D. (1983). *Neuropsychological assessment* (2nd Ed.). New York: Oxford.

Liberman, R. P. (Ed.) (1988). *Psychiatric rehabilitation of chronic mental patients*. Washington, D. C.: American Psychiatric Association.

Luria, A. R. (1966). *Higher cortical functions in man*. New York: Basic Books.

Luria, A. R. (1973). *The working brain*. New York: Basic Books.

Meier, M., Benton, A., & Diller, L. (Eds.) (1987). *Neuropsychological rehabilitation*. New York: Guilford.

Poon, L. W., et al.. (Eds.) (1986). *The handbook of clinical memory assessment of older adults*. Washington, D. C.: American Psychological Assocation.

Prigatano, G. P. (1986). *Neuropsychological rehabilitation after head injury*. Baltimore: Johns Hopkins University.

Sohlberg, M. M., & Mateer, C. A. (1987). Effectiveness of an attention-training program. *Journal of Clinical and Experimental Neuropsychology*, 9, 117–130.

Spaulding, W. D., Storms, L., Goodrich, V., & Sullivan, M. (1986). Applications of experimental psychopathology in psychiatric rehabilitation. *Schizophrenia Bulletin*, 12, 560–577.

Sternberg, R. J. (1985). *Beyond IQ*. New York: Cambridge.

Sternberg, R. J. (1988). *The triarchic mind*. New York: Viking.

Sternberg, R. J. (1990). *Metaphors of mind*. New York: Cambridge.

Sternberg, J., & Smith, E. E. (Eds.). (1986). *The psychology of human thought*. New York: Cambridge.

Sternberg, R. J., & Wagner, R. K. (Eds.) (1987). *Practical intelligence*. New York: Cambridge.

Stuve, P., Erickson, R. C., & Spaulding, W. D. (1991). Cognitive rehabilitation: The next step in psychological rehabilitation. *Psychosocial Rehabilitation Journal*, 15, 9–26.

Townes, B. D., et al. (1985). Neurobehavioral approach to classification of psychiatric patients using a competency model. *Journal of Consulting and Clinical Psychology*, 53, 33–42.

Trexler, L. E. (Ed.) (1982). *Cognitive rehabilitation: Conceptualization and intervention*. New York: Plenum.

Willis, S. L., & Schaie, K. W. (1989). Practical intelligence in later adulthood. In R. J. Sternberg & R. K. Wagner (Eds.), *Practical intelligence* (pp. 236–268). New York: Cambridge.

Wilson, B. A. (1987). *Rehabilitation of memory.* New York: Guilford.

Yozawitz, A. (1986). Applied neuropsychology in a psychiatric center. In I. Grant & K. M. Adams (Eds.), *Neuropsychological assessment of neuropsychiatric disorders* (pp. 121–146). New York: Oxford.

•4•

Cognitive Prerequisites of Skill Acquisition in Schizophrenia: Bridging Micro- and Macro-Levels of Processing

Robert S. Kern and Michael F. Green

Training schizophrenic and other psychiatric patients in specialized skills has won wider acceptance over the past 10 to 15 years. Unidimensional treatment strategies, i.e., pharmacological interventions alone, have been shown to be effective for management of symptoms, but such strategies do not teach patients new skills that could help them maintain an independent or semi-independent status in the community. Hence, many psychiatric facilities have added skills training programs. Most studies have shown skills training to be generally effective, but the factors behind its success have been largely unexplored. The present chapter will examine the relationship of cognitive factors to skills training.

Skills Training Programs

Skills training programs were developed to equip adult psychiatric patients with self-help skills. The primary goal is to provide patients with the means to live semi-independently and to achieve greater control over their behavior. Participants are taught independent-living skills, including interpersonal problem solving, socialization, and medication and symptom management. Several studies have shown improved social functioning, fewer relapses, and less time in the hospital for patients who engaged in skills training programs (Bellack et al., 1984; Benton & Schroeder, 1990; Finch & Wallace, 1977; Hogarty et al., 1986; Liberman et al., 1985; Lukoff et al., 1986). Furthermore, the durability of these gains has been shown for up to two years following discharge (Liberman, Mueser & Wallace, 1986; Wallace & Liberman, 1985).

Skills training programs are typically divided into areas of specific content, e.g., interpersonal skills or medication management. The methods of training combine didactic instruction with applied principles of learning theory. A typical training session may include classroom instruction, modeling, corrective feedback, and behavioral rehearsal. Videotaped vignettes may supplement the didactic component. Training is provided in a highly interactive small group format, taught by one or two trained instructors. The training groups generally meet daily for one to two hours, with module completion requiring between four and eight months. Upon completion of training, each individual demonstrates competence in the designated skill area by completing an examination that measures knowledge of content, skill acquisition via role playing, knowledge about resource management, and problem-solving ability.

Initially, studies attempted to show that psychiatric patients who participated in skills training improved more in overall functioning than did patients who had not received skills training. These studies yielded promising results that helped to establish skills training as a viable form of treatment. However, they did not explain the observed individual variability within the programs. Given the method of instruction in skills training, it is reasonable to expect that individual differences in cognitive processing ability might be related to performance differences.

Cognition

Functionally, cognition is defined as "all processes by which sensory input is transformed, reduced, elaborated, stored, recovered, and used" (Neisser, 1967). It includes such functions as attention, perception, sensation, problem-solving ability, language, visuo-spatial ability, and concept formation (Glass, Holyoak & Santa, 1979).

Cognition is frequently conceptualized by a micro- to macro-level scale that attempts to encompass the range of cognitive functioning. At the molecular, or micro-level, cognitive processes are represented primarily as unitary functions, and may be conceptualized as the building blocks for higher macro-level behaviors. An example of a function at this level would be early visual processing, a sensory-perceptual function. Molar cognitive processes, which are more complex, represent the integration of specific cognitive processes that operate at molecular levels (Ben-Yishay & Diller, 1983; Reed et al., 1991; Spaulding et al., 1986). Social behavior is an example of a macro-level function because it requires the integration of various cognitive functions. Competency in social behavior requires intact functioning of attention, perception, language (expressive and receptive), and executive abilities.

Where does skills training fall on the continuum of micro- to macro-levels of cognitive functioning? Skills training is probably best conceptualized as a macro-level process because successful performance requires proficiency across several domains. The individual must be able to demonstrate content knowledge, perform role-playing activities, demonstrate knowledge about social and informational resources, and problem-solve. Within this framework, which cognitive functions might show the strongest association with success in skills training? One might predict that the strongest association would be with measures of attention, memory, and verbal ability as opposed to measures of nonverbal processing (e.g., visuo-spatial ability), since the former would appear necessary for the structured didactic setting.

Given the prominent role of skills training programs in psychiatric rehabilitation, it will become critical to identify cognitive factors associated with successful outcome. Investigations must include: (1) areas of cognitive dysfunction in schizophrenia; (2) preliminary studies of cognitive functioning and skills training; (3) generalization issues; and (4) directions for future skills training.

AREAS OF COGNITIVE DYSFUNCTION IN SCHIZOPHRENIA

A number of studies have identified cognitive deficits in schizophrenia across a variety of domains, including memory, attention, language, and frontal systems functioning (Calev, Venables & Monk, 1983; Erickson & Binder, 1986; Flor-Henry, 1976; Goldberg et al., 1987; Goldstein, 1986; Gur, 1978; Koh & Kayton, 1974; Kolb & Whishaw, 1983; McKenna et al., 1990; Oltmanns & Neale, 1975; Weinberger, Berman & Zec, 1986). The following sections briefly review the results from a few representative studies in this area.

1. *Verbal Memory.* Deficits in memory and learning have been consistently reported in schizophrenic patients, and these deficits appear to be more severe than in other areas of cognitive functioning (Saykin et al., 1991). Memory functioning may be conceptually divided into four stages: perception, encoding, storage, and retrieval. Dysfunction anywhere along the stages of memory

processing may adversely affect performance at a subsequent stage (Sacuzzo & Braff, 1981). For example, dysfunction at the encoding stage may affect storage or retrieval processes.

In the case of schizophrenia, several investigators have suggested that a deficit exists in the encoding stage and that it subsequently affects retrieval (Kay, 1982; Yu & Johnson, 1979). Deficits in encoding may be related to inefficiencies in organization. Schizophrenic patients may underutilize semantic information, attending instead to less salient stimulus features (e.g., physical characteristics) or irrelevant stimuli (e.g., distractors). Since recall relies on previously formed associations, it has been hypothesized that schizophrenic patients' difficulties in recall result from deficiencies in forming meaningful associations (Kay, 1982). In other words, the poor recall observed in many schizophrenic patients may be related to their underutilization of salient stimulus features for categorization during the encoding stage. Recently, Wallace et al. (1991) found that schizophrenic patients were able to recall successfully a large number of unrelated words when they were required initially to process the words either phonetically (by providing a word that rhymes) or semantically (by providing a word that means the same). These results suggest that when directed to use specific strategies, schizophrenic patients show recall abilities that approach normal levels of functioning.

Consistent with an encoding deficit in schizophrenia is the finding that schizophrenic patients typically show far better performance on recognition tasks than on recall tasks (Calev et al., 1983; Calev, 1984; Koh, 1978). This finding has been reported by a number of investigators (Bauman & Murray, 1968; Magaro & Page, 1982; Nachmani & Cohen, 1969). Inefficiencies in the organization of material during the encoding stage are likely to have an adverse effect on recall, but not necessarily on recognition. The reason is that recall, being a more active process, is enhanced by association properties. The number and strength of previously formed associations is related to recall performance. Recognition, on the other hand, is a more passive process and places less demand on encoding efficiency.

Goldberg and Weinberger (1988) found differential levels of performance on recall and recognition within their sample of schizophrenic patients. The memory measure in the study used a selective reminding procedure. The schizophrenic group showed minor gains in the number of recalled words over the 12 learning trials, although the slope of the learning curve was inferior to that obtained by normal controls. Assessment of *recognition* abilities, by contrast, indicated that schizophrenic patients showed gains similar to those of normal controls.

Similarly, Koh, Kayton, and Berry (1973) found that schizophrenic patients performed better on tests of recognition than on recall. They suggested that schizophrenic patients have difficulty in organizing or "chunking" material into meaningful units. This limitation taxes the operating capacity of short-term memory, thereby reducing the amount of information that can be remembered at one time.

The selective pattern of deficits in memory functioning is inconsistent with a generalized deterioration model (i.e., one that postulates pervasive deficits across all cognitive domains; Flor-Henry, 1976) and more closely resembles the pattern of deficits seen in a specific deficit syndrome (Calev et al., 1983). Some investigators liken the memory deficits of schizophrenic patients to those observed in alcoholic Korsakoff's disorder (McKenna et al., 1990). The most oft-noted signs in both are impaired learning, rapid forgetting, and better performance on remote memory measures than on learning measures. Though both disorders share similarities in the memory deficits, certain inconsistencies remain (e.g., the lack of an amnesic gradient for remote memory in schizophrenic patients; Calev, Berlin & Lerer, 1987).

2. *Attention.* Attentional deficits have been frequently documented in schizophrenic patients (Bleuler, 1950 [1911]; McGhie & Chapman, 1961; Orzack & Kornetsky, 1966; Walker, 1981). Attentional processes may be divided conceptually into areas of selective and sustained attention. Selective attention refers to the ability to attend to stimuli in the presence of a distractor; it may be measured using a test such as the Digit Span Distractibility Test (Oltmanns & Neale, 1975), in which the subject recalls a string of numbers under distracting and under neutral conditions. On the other hand, sustained attention refers to the ability to maintain performance levels over time, as measured by a test such as the Continuous Performance Test (Rosvold et al., 1956). The two constructs of interest for the Continuous Performance Test are vigilance level, or the overall ability to distinguish between target and noise, and vigilance decrement, or the amount of change in performance between the beginning and the end of the test.

Oltmanns & Neale (1977) provided evidence of a deficit in selective attention in schizophrenia using the Digit Span Distractibility Test. They reported that schizophrenic patients performed worse than controls under both neutral and distracting conditions of the test; moreover, the schizophrenic patients in their sample showed greater difficulty than controls under the distracting condition for longer digit strings. The two conditions were equated for level of difficulty and internal consistency. It was suggested that these findings reflect a selective deficit that goes beyond micro-level sensory encoding. This type of dysfunction may be related to deficiencies in organization. More specifically, the organizing capabilities of schizophrenic patients may be adversely affected by a failure in transforming information into meaningful "chunks." With respect to the relationship between selective attention and symptomatology, Green and Walker (1986) found that positive-symptom schizophrenic patients were more susceptible to distraction than negative-symptom patients as evidenced by greater performance decrement on the distraction condition of the Digit Span Distractibility Test.

Other procedures used to assess selective attention include dichotic listening tasks. Under such conditions, schizophrenic patients typically make more errors of omission than comparison groups in verbal shadowing of the relevant message (Hemsley & Richardson, 1980; Payne, Hochberg & Hawks, 1970; Rappaport, 1967; Schneider, 1976; Wishner & Wahl, 1974). These results suggest that schizophrenic patients may also be more susceptible to distraction than other patient groups. Offering further support for a distraction hypothesis, investigators have reported that schizophrenic patients frequently make intrusion errors, confusing the relevant and irrelevant messages (Spring et al., 1989).

Not surprisingly, some investigators have found that the deficits in selective attention are not specific to schizophrenia. Everett, Laplante, and Thomas (1989) compared schizophrenic and nonschizophrenic (depressed) inpatients on the Stroop Color-Word Test, which can be considered a measure of selective attention. They found that schizophrenic subjects did not differ from depressed patients in their ability to attend selectively to a particular feature of a stimulus.

Deficits in sustained attention have been observed in schizophrenic patients in both clinical and experimental settings. A majority of the evidence concerning sustained attention suggests that schizophrenic patients differ from normal individuals only in certain specific aspects of sustained attention. Differences between schizophrenic groups and controls have been found for vigilance level, but not for vigilance decrement, on the Continuous Performance Test (Cornblatt, Lenzenweger & Erlenmeyer-Kimling, 1989; Green, Nuechterlein & Gaier, in press; Nuechterlein, 1983; Orzack & Kornetsky, 1966).

In summary, several studies have shown deficits in selective and sustained attention in schizophrenic patients. The deficits appear to be related to difficulties in organization and distractibility. Furthermore, there is support for varying levels of attentional ability within schizophrenic patients, ranging from near normal to impaired ranges.

3. *Language.* Several investigators have speculated that the disorders of thought and language in schizophrenia are related to dysfunction of the left hemisphere, primarily in the temporal region (Flor-Henry, 1976; Gur, 1978; Gur et al., 1987; Suddath et al., 1989). However, there has been some difference of opinion as to whether the disorders of language in schizophrenia are primary, i.e., sharing the neurological properties of aphasic syndromes, or whether they are manifestations of an underlying thought disorder. Schizophrenic patients may show thought disorders such as circumstantiality, tangentiality, derailment, loosening of associations, incoherent speech, or poverty of content. On the other hand, some patients exhibit symptoms more typified by aphasic syndromes, e.g., paraphasic output (use of incorrect words that are approximations of the correct word). When Andreasen and Grove (1979) compared schizophrenic patients and manic patients to patients with Wernicke's aphasia, they found the language deficits in the schizophrenic group to be representative of a mild language disorder. Sixteen percent of the schizophrenic patients showed marked speech incoherence. Language disturbances in schizophrenia have also been associated with greater cognitive compromise and longer duration of illness (Silverberg-Shalev et al., 1981).

4. *Executive Functions.* Assessment of frontal systems functioning has revealed dysfunction in schizophrenia manifested by difficulties in abstraction, sequential organization, fluency, and planning. Behaviorally, some schizophrenic patients show a lack of motivation and drive. Others demonstrate impulse control problems, and some may engage in bizarre behavior, e.g., fecal smearing. A test frequently used to assess frontal systems functioning is the Wisconsin Card Sorting Test (Heaton, 1981). This measure assesses cognitive flexibility and concept formation. Schizophrenic patients have consis-

tently performed poorly on this test (Bellack et al., 1989; Braff et al., 1989; Goldberg et al., 1987). Further support for executive dysfunction in schizophrenia has been found in activation studies that have shown reduced blood flow to the dorsolateral prefrontal cortex during tasks that "activate" those regions (Berman, Zec & Weinberger, 1986; Weinberger, Berman & Zec, 1986).

PRELIMINARY STUDIES OF COGNITIVE FUNCTIONING AND SKILLS TRAINING

Because of the diversity and range of cognitive processes, it is reasonable to expect that various processing stages would show a differential relationship to skills training. For example, measurement of early visual processing speed may provide important information about patients' processing capacity and the speed at which information can be effectively incorporated. On the other hand, assessment at a more intermediate level, i.e., verbal memory, may provide information about processing ability similar to that utilized during skills training.

In three separate studies at UCLA-Camarillo State Hospital and one study at Eastern Pennsylvania Psychiatric Institute, the preliminary results stimulate hypotheses about the relationship between information processing and skills training. Bowen et al. (1990), using a cross-sectional design, investigated the relationship between cognitive factors and skills training (basic learning skills, problem-solving skills, and social skills). Subjects were administered a brief battery of information processing measures that included the Continuous Performance Test, a degraded-stimulus version of the same test, the Digit Span Distractibility Test, and the Span of Apprehension Test. Outcome measures were drawn from the Medication Management Module (Liberman, 1986) and the Assessment of Interpersonal Problem-Solving Skills (AIPSS; Donahoe et al., 1984; 1990). The measures of early visual processing, sustained vigilance, and distractibility were successful predictors of skills training outcome in a group of schizophrenic inpatients. Similarly, Corrigan et al. (1991) reported that freedom from distractibility was predictive of skills training ability on the Medication Management Module and the AIPSS in a comparable group of psychiatric inpatients. However, Corrigan et al. also found verbal memory to be highly correlated with social problem-solving ability (AIPSS) and skills training outcome (Medication Management Module). It should be noted that the study by Bowen et al. did not include a measure of verbal memory. Kern, Green, and Satz (1990) found that verbal memory, freedom from distractibility, and vigilance decrement predicted skills training success (basic learning skills) on the Medication Management Module. The latter study, which used a longitudinal design, found that cognitive measures tended to be better at predicting ability before skills training than posttest outcome. Finally, Mueser et al. (1991) found that poor memory functioning was predictive of social skills impairments and slower rates of skills improvement. Interestingly, this group also examined symptomatology as a predictor of social skills training success and found little association between the two. These four studies offer some initial support for the hypothesis that cognitive deficits act as rate-limiting factors in skills acquisition. The studies of Kern et al., Corrigan et al., and Mueser et al. suggest that verbal memory may be particularly relevant to skills acquisition.

Consider the range of cognitive functions that were found to correlate with success in skills training. The measures of cognitive functioning included in these studies covered micro- to macro-levels of information processing. The study by Bowen et al. suggests that micro-levels of information processing can offer predictive utility in skills training. Span of Apprehension, a test of visual search and iconic readout (a micro-level process), strongly predicts skill acquisition on the Medication Management Module. Perhaps the ability to register multiple bits of information is necessary for didactic training. In general, though, intermediate levels of information processing have more frequently been found to be predictive of skills training success. Specifically, cognitive measures of verbal memory and freedom from distractibility, and perhaps of vigilance with high processing load, have been reported to be successful predictors of skills ability and acquisition (Kern et al., 1990; Corrigan et al., 1991; Mueser et al., 1991). The Kern et al. and Corrigan et al. studies used the same measure of verbal memory, the Rey Auditory Verbal Learning Test (Rey, 1964), and Mueser et al. used the Wechsler Memory Scale. Interestingly, the studies by Bowen et al., Kern et al., and Corrigan et al. all agreed on the predictive utility of a measure of serial recall and selective attention, the Digit Span Distractibility Test. These cognitive functions, which fall at the intermediate level of information processing, may represent, more than other cognitive functions, those abilities necessary for successful performance on measures of skill attainment.

Based on these preliminary findings, it appears that verbal memory, freedom from distractibility, and possibly visual vigilance and iconic readout are related to skills training ability. Preliminary evidence indicates involvement of primarily intermediate levels of information processing. Furthermore, these findings suggest that certain patients may be affected by rate-limiting factors that impede or prevent their ability to process information and acquire new self-help skills.

Generalization Issues

Targeting intervention at micro-level processes rests on the assumption that remediation at elementary processing levels will lead to changes in more complex, higher-level processes. For example, remediating attentional deficits will lead to improved social behavior. Except for a brief period of exploration with some notable results in the 1960s and 1970s, little attention has been paid to the role of remediating cognition in schizophrenia. Though it has been shown that macro-level psychosocial interventions, e.g., skills training programs, serve to improve the functioning of psychiatric patients by stabilizing symptoms, reducing recidivism, and reducing the number of hospitalizations, it has not been shown that these macro-level psychosocial interventions can improve elementary, micro-level cognitive functions as well. In fact, the validity of this type of downward generalization, from macro-level intervention to micro-level cognitive process, has been largely unexplored (Spaulding et al., 1986; Spring & Ravden, 1992). On the other hand, there is some empirical evidence that would justify remediation efforts at the elementary, micro-level cognitive processing stage with the aim of improving complex, macro-level behaviors.

Wagner (1968) trained schizophrenic subjects on attending and abstracting responses. During attention training, subjects were shown a number of slides and then asked to select the stimulus (e.g., simple geometrical figure) that correctly matched the stimulus shown. Abstraction training followed a similar procedure. During abstraction training, subjects attempted to select the stimulus that correctly matched a previously shown stimulus in terms of a common attribute (e.g., shape). Wagner found that performance could be improved under conditions of contingent reinforcement. Training on these micro-level tasks improved performance on higher-level intellectual tasks, thus providing support for upward generalization. Training on the attending and abstracting tasks did not lead to differential improvement on the intellectual measures, however. Wagner concluded that these findings argue against a deficit theory that posits an inability to perform select functions. He concluded that attending and abstracting responses indeed exist in the repertoire of the schizophrenic patient, but occur with less frequency than other behaviors.

One of the more impressive displays of generalization across tasks was demonstrated in a series of studies by Meichenbaum (1966, 1969; Meichenbaum & Cameron, 1973). In one study, contingent reinforcement programs used social and token reinforcers. The primary aim was to improve level of abstraction, but the effects of the intervention subsequently generalized to decreasing deviant verbalizations as well. Furthermore, patients were found to engage spontaneously in self-instruction, telling themselves to pay attention and speak coherently. The second study, which targeted self-instruction, attempted to improve patients' ability to self-instruct through the use of cognitive modeling and rehearsal procedures. These early efforts at showing generalizability effects were promising, though not always replicated (Margolis & Shemberg, 1976).

Recently, a few training programs have attempted to maximize treatment effectiveness by combining cognitive exercises and social skills training. Brenner's Integrated Psychological Treatment (IPT) is based on the potential efficacy of training generalization (Brenner, 1989). This program includes components designed to train psychiatric patients in areas of both cognitive and social functioning. The cognitive component includes training of intermediate to complex cognitive processes. In a study examining the effects of cognitive and social skills training on psychotic symptoms, Brenner (1989) found that patients showed improved cognition and reduced symptomatology following participation in the program.

Similarly, Kraemer, Zinner, and Moller (1989) studied the differential effects of cognitive therapy and social skills training on cognition and on psychopathology. Outcome measures were collected pre- and posttraining and at a one-half-year follow-up. Cognitive therapy trained patients on exercises of perception and problem-solving ability modeled after Brenner's IPT program. These authors found that both cognitive therapy and social skills training showed mild, but similar, gains in cognitive functioning.

To assess treatment effectiveness, measures were collected on negative symptoms, psychotic symptoms, and social functioning. Cognitive therapy was found to be superior to social skills training in alleviating negative symptoms, and the gains stabilized over time. Less disturbance was noted in such areas as language and perception, and patients were found to be less anxious and to show fewer signs of overstimulation. In terms of reducing psychotic symptoms, both cognitive therapy and social skills training were effective at showing mild improvement. The gains in the cognitive therapy group were not maintained over time, however. Finally, the social functioning of the cognitive therapy group improved more than in the social skills training group, though improved functioning was noted by patients in both groups. Patients in the cognitive therapy group noted that they felt less anxious about receiving criticism and about being involved in interpersonal contact, whereas patients in the social skills training group stated that they were better equipped to initiate contact with other persons. Overall, cognitive therapy was found to be superior to social skills training at improving patient functioning; however, Kraemer et al. affirmed the value of social skills training and suggested that a combination of the two would be optimal for future rehabilitation programs.

Olbrich and Mussgay (1990) employed training procedures that emphasized rehearsal. During training, subjects practiced performing tasks of medium complexity (similar to the type of tasks described by Kraemer, e.g., reasoning and concept formation, visual and verbal recall). It was found that training on these measures improved performance on tasks of comparable complexity (e.g., embedded figures test), but not on micro-level tasks. Hence, their findings offered support for the usefulness of cognitive interventions only to improve performance across tasks of similar complexity, a type of lateral generalization.

In general, the small number of studies in the area of generalizability offer some promise that training psychiatric patients on cognitive exercises can promote performance in other areas of functioning. It appears that for upward generalization to be maximally effective, the cognitive training task needs to be functionally similar to a component of the macro-level outcome behavior.

Directions for Future Skills Training Programs

Results from these and similar studies support the development of enriched treatment programs designed to enhance suspected processing deficits. The most promising possibility may be comprehensive training programs that combine pharmacological intervention with skills training modules that employ cognitive assessment and remediation as well as behavioral-based instruction. For such integrated training programs, the assessment of information-processing capabilities becomes an essential component. Early detection of information-processing deficits can be used to help those patients who would otherwise be left to struggle in a typical training environment. Once identified, these disadvantaged patients can be targeted for cognitive remediation. Enhancing the ability of psychiatric patients to acquire information has obvious implications. For example, if the attention and memory abilities of these patients can be improved, then perhaps their ability to acquire instructional material may be enhanced as well. An alternative to this type of program would be one geared to tailoring training tasks to meet the processing limitations of individual patients.

Similarly designed programs offer the hope of successfully providing independent living skills to more psychiatric patients. The need for improved skills training programs to more effectively treat psychiatric patients with a variety of cognitive disturbances should be clear. A number of studies have shown that providing independent living skills to psychiatric patients serves a protective function, preventing relapse and reducing number of hospital admissions. Placing greater emphasis on prevention of psychiatric relapse is likely to result in personal, economic, and social benefits.

References

Andreasen, N. C., & Grove, W. (1979). The relationship between schizophrenic language, manic language and aphasia. In J. Gruzelier & P. Flor-Henry (Eds.), *Hemisphere asymmetries in function psychopathology.* Amsterdam: Elsevier.

Bauman, E., & Murray, D. J. (1968). Recognition versus recall in schizophrenia. *Canadian Journal of Psychology,* 22, 18–25.

Bellack, A. S., Mueser, K. T., Morrison, R. L., Tierney, B. A., & Podell, K. (1989). Remediation of cognitive deficits in schizophrenia. *American Journal of Psychiatry,* 147, 1650–1655.

Bellack, A. S., Turner, S. M., Hersen, M., & Luber, R. F. (1984). An examination of the efficacy of social skills training for chronic psychiatric patients. *Hospital and Community Psychiatry,* 35, 1023–1028.

Benton, M. K., & Schroeder, H. E. (1990). Social skills training with schizophrenics: A meta-analytic evaluation. *Journal of Consulting and Clinical Psychology,* 58, 741–747.

Ben-Yishay, Y., & Diller, L. (1983). Cognitive remediation. In M. Rosenthal, E. R. Griffith, M. R. Bond, & J. D. Miller (Eds.), *Rehabilitation of the head-injured adult* (pp. 367–379). Philadelphia: F. A. Davis.

Berman, K. F., Zec, R. F., & Weinberger, D. R. (1986). Physiologic dysfunction of dorsolateral prefrontal cortex in schizophrenia: II. Role of neuroleptic treatment, attention, and mental effort. *Archives of General Psychiatry,* 43, 126–135.

Bleuler, E. (1950 [1911]). *Dementia praecox, or the group of schizophrenias.* Trans. 1950 by J. Zinkin. New York: International Universities Press.

Bowen, L., Wallace, C. J., Glynn, S. M., Nuechterlein, K. H., Lutzker, J. R., & Kuehnel, T. G. (1989). Relationships among schizophrenic patients on attentional skills, social problem-solving skills, and performance in psychoeducational rehabilitation tasks. Paper presented at the 23rd annual meeting of the Association for the Advancement of Behavior Therapy, Washington, D. C.

Brenner, H. D. (1989). The treatment of basic psychological dysfunctions from a systemic point of view. *British Journal of Psychiatry,* 155 (suppl. 5), 74–83.

Braff, D. L., Butler, R. B., Jenkins, M., & Geyer, M. A. (1989). Wisconsin card sorting performance in schizophrenia: Neurophysiological correlates. Paper presented at the annual meeting of the American College of Neuropsychopharmacology, Maui, Hawaii.

Calev, A. (1984). Recall and recognition in chronic nondemented schizophrenics: Use of matched tasks. *Journal of Abnormal Psychology,* 93, 172–177.

Calev, A., Berlin, H., & Lerer, B. (1987). Remote and recent memory in long-hospitalized chronic schizophrenics. *Biological Psychiatry,* 22, 79–85.

Calev, A., Venables, P. H., & Monk, A. F. (1983). Evidence for distinct verbal memory pathologies in severely and mildly disturbed schizophrenics. *Schizophrenia Bulletin,* 19, 247–264.

Cornblatt, B., Lenzenweger, M. F., & Erlenmeyer-Kimling, L. (1989). The continuous performance test, identical pairs version: II. Contrasting attentional profiles in schizophrenic and depressed patients. *Psychiatry Research,* 29, 65–85.

Corrigan, P. W., Wallace, C. J., Green, M. F., & Schade, M. L. (1991). Cognition and social functioning in schizophrenia. Paper presented at the annual meeting of the American Psychiatric Association, New Orleans, La.

Donahoe, C. P., Carter, M. J., Bloem, W. D., Hirsch, G. L., Laasi, N., & Wallace, C. J. (1990). Assessment of interpersonal problem-solving skills. *Psychiatry,* 53, 329–339.

Donahoe, C. P., Carter, M. J., Bloem, W. D., & Leff, G. Y. (1984). Assessment of interpersonal problem solving skills. Unpublished test manual.

Erickson, R. C., & Binder, L. M. (1986). Cognitive deficits among functionally psychotic patients: A rehabilitative perspective. *Journal of Clinical and Experimental Neuropsychology,* 8, 257–274.

Everett, J., Laplante, L., & Thomas, J. (1989). The selective attention deficit in schizophrenia: Limited resources or cognitive fatigue? *Journal of Nervous and Mental Disease,* 177, 735–738.

Finch, B. E., & Wallace, C. J. (1977). Successful interpersonal skills training with schizophrenic inpatients. *Journal of Consulting and Clinical Psychology,* 45, 885–890.

Flor-Henry, P. (1976). Lateralized temporal lymbic dysfunction and psychopathology. *Annals of the New York Academy of Sciences,* 280, 777–795.

Glass, A. L., Holyoak, K. J., & Santa, J. L. (1979). *Cognition.* Reading, Mass.: Addison-Wesley Publishing Company.

Goldberg, T. E., & Weinberger, D. R. (1988). Probing prefrontal function in schizophrenia with neuropsychological paradigms. *Schizophrenia Bulletin,* 14, 179–183.

Goldberg, T. E., Weinberger, D. R., Pliskin, N. H., Berman, K. F., & Podd, M. H. (1989). Recall memory deficit in schizophrenia: A possible manifestation of prefrontal dysfunction. *Schizophrenia Research,* 2, 251–257.

Goldstein, G. (1986). The neuropsychology of schizophrenia. In I. Grant & K. M. Adams (Eds.), *Neuropsychological assessment of neuropsychiatric disorders* (pp. 147–171). New York: Oxford University Press.

Green, M. F., Nuechterlein, K. H., & Gaier, D. J. (In press). Sustained and selective attention in schizophrenia. *Progress in Experimental Personality and Psychopathology Research.*

Green, M. F., & Walker, E. (1986). Attentional performance in positive- and negative-symptom schizophrenia. *Journal of Nervous and Mental Disease,* 174, 208–213.

Gur, R. E. (1978). Left hemisphere dysfunction and left hemisphere overactivation in schizophrenia. *Journal of Abnormal Psychology,* 87, 226–238.

Gur, R. E., Resnick, S. M., Alavi, A., Gur, R. C., Caroff, S., Dann, R., Silver, F., Saykin, A. J., Chawluk, J. B., Kushner, M., & Reivich, M. (1987). Regional brain function in schizophrenia: I. A positron emission tomography study. *Archives of General Psychiatry,* 44, 119–125.

Heaton, R. K. (1981). Wisconsin Card Sorting Test manual. Odessa, Fla.: Psychological Assessment Resources.

Hemsley, D. R., & Richardson, P. H. (1980). Shadowing by context in schizophrenia. *Journal of Nervous and Mental Disease,* 168, 141–145.

Hogarty, G. E., Anderson, C. M., Reiss, D. J., Kornblith, S. J., Greenwald, D. P., Javna, C. D., & Madonia, M. J. (1986). Family psychoeducation, social skills training, and maintenance chemotherapy in the aftercare treatment of schizophrenia. *Archives of General Psychiatry,* 43, 633–642.

Kay, S. R. (1982). Conceptual disorder in schizophrenia as a function of encoding orientation. *Journal of Nervous and Mental Disease,* 170, 154–163.

Kern, R. S., Green, M. F., & Satz, P. (1990, December). Neuropsychological predictors of outcome in skills training. Paper presented at the 5th annual meeting of the Society for Research in Psychopathology, Boulder, Colo.

Koh, S. D. (1978). Remembering of verbal materials by schizophrenic young adults. In S. Schwartz (Ed.), *Language and cognition in schizophrenia* (pp. 55–99). Hillsdale, N.J.: Erlbaum.

Koh, S. D., & Kayton, L. (1974). Memorization of "unrelated" word strings by young nonpsychotic schizophrenics. *Journal of Abnormal Psychology,* 83, 14–22.

Koh, S. D., Kayton, L., & Berry, R. (1973). Mnemonic organization in young nonpsychotic schizophrenics. *Journal of Abnormal Psychology,* 81, 299–310.

Kolb, B., & Whishaw, I. Q. (1983). Performance of schizophrenic patients on tests sensitive to left or right frontal, temporal, or parietal function in neurological patients. *Journal of Nervous and Mental Disease,* 171, 435–443.

Kraemer, S., Zinner, H. J., & Moller, H. J. (1989, October). Cognitive therapy and social skills training in chronic schizophrenic patients. Paper presented at the World Congress of Psychiatry.

Liberman, R. P. (1986). *The Medication Management Module.* Camarillo, Calif.: UCLA Clinical Research Center for Schizophrenia and Psychiatric Rehabilitation.

Liberman, R. P., Massel, H. K., Mosk, M. D., & Wong, S. E. (1985). Social skills training for chronic mental patients. *Hospital and Community Psychiatry,* 36, 396–403.

Liberman, R. P., Mueser, K. T., & Wallace, C. J. (1986). Social skills training for schizophrenic individuals at risk for relapse. *American Journal of Psychiatry,* 143, 523–526.

Liberman, R. P., Nuechterlein, K. H., & Wallace, C. W. (1982). Social skills training and the nature of schizophrenia. In J. Curran & P. Monti (Eds.), *Social skills training: A practical handbook for assessment and treatment.* New York: Guilford Press.

Lukoff, D., Wallace, C. J., Liberman, R. P., & Burke, K. (1986). A holistic program for chronic schizophrenic patients. *Schizophrenia Bulletin,* 12, 274–282.

McGhie, A., & Chapman, J. (1961). Disorders of attention and perception in early schizophrenia. *British Journal of Medical Psychology,* 34, 103–117.

McKenna, P. J., Tamlyn, D., Lund, C. E., Mortimer, A. M., Hammond, S., & Baddeley, A. D. (1990). Amnesic syndrome in schizophrenia. *Psychological Medicine,* 20, 967–972.

Magaro, P. A., & Page, J. (1982). Icon thresholds in paranoid and non-paranoid schizophrenics. *British Journal of Clinical Psychology,* 21, 213–219.

Margolis, R. B., & Shemberg, K. M. (1976). Cognitive self-instruction in process and reactive schizophrenics: A failure to replicate. *Behavior Therapy,* 7, 668–671.

Meichenbaum, D. H. (1966). Effects of social reinforcement on the level of abstraction in schizophrenics. *Journal of Abnormal Psychology,* 71, 354–362.

Meichenbaum, D. H. (1969). The effects of instructions and reinforcement on thinking and language behavior of schizophrenics. *Behavior Research and Therapy,* 7, 101–114.

Meichenbaum, D. H., & Cameron, R. (1973). Training schizophrenics to talk to themselves: A means of developing attentional controls. *Behavior Therapy,* 4, 515–534.

Mueser, K. T., Bellack, A. S., Douglas, M. S., & Wade, J. H. (1991). Prediction of social skill acquisition in schizophrenic and major affective disorder patients from memory and symptomatology. *Psychiatry Research*, 37, 281–296.

Nachmani, G., & Cohen, B. D. (1969). Recall and recognition free learning in schizophrenics. *Journal of Abnormal Psychology*, 74, 511–516.

Neisser, U. (1967). *Cognitive Psychology*. New York: Appleton-Century-Crofts.

Nuechterlein, K. H. (1983). Signal detection in vigilance tasks and behavioral attributes among offspring of schizophrenic mothers and among hyperactive children. *Journal of Abnormal Psychology*, 92, 4–28.

Nuechterlein, K. H., & Dawson, M. E. (1984). Information processing and attentional functioning in the developmental course of schizophrenia. *Schizophrenia Bulletin*, 10, 160–203.

Olbrich, R., & Mussgay, L. (1990). Reduction of schizophrenic deficits by cognitive training: An evaluative study. *European Archives of Psychiatry and Neurological Science*, 239, 366–369.

Oltmanns, T. F., & Neale, J. M. (1975). Schizophrenic performance when distractors are present: Attentional deficit or differential task difficulty? *Journal of Abnormal Psychology*, 84, 205–209.

Orzack, M. H., & Kornetsky, C. (1966). Attention dysfunction in chronic schizophrenia. *Archives of General Psychiatry*, 14, 323–326.

Payne, R. W., Hochberg, A. C., & Hawks, D. V. (1970). Dichotic stimulation as a method of assessing disorder of attention in over-inclusive schizophrenic patients. *Journal of Abnormal Psychology*, 76, 185–193.

Rappaport, M. (1967). Competing voice messages: Effect of message load and drugs on the ability of acute schizophrenics to attend. *Archives of General Psychiatry*, 17, 97–103.

Reed, D., Sullivan, M., Penn, D. L., Stuve, P., & Spaulding, W. (1991). Assessment and treatment of cognitive impairments in psychiatric rehabilitation. Unpublished manuscript.

Rey, A. (1964). *L'examen clinique en psychologie*. Paris: Presses Universitaires de France.

Rosvold, H. E., Mirsky, A., Sarason, I., Bransome, E. D., Jr., & Beck, L. H. (1956). A continuous performance test of brain damage. *Journal of Consulting Psychology*, 20, 343–350.

Sacuzzo, D. P., & Braff, D. L. (1981). Early information processing deficit in schizophrenia. *Archives of General Psychiatry*, 38, 175–179.

Saykin, A. J., Gur, R. C., Gur, R. E., Mozley, D., Mozley, L. H., Resnick, S. M., Kester, B., & Stafiniak, P. (1991). Neuropsychological function in schizophrenia. *Archives of General Psychiatry*, 48, 618–624.

Schneider, S. J. (1976). Selective attention in schizophrenia. *Journal of Abnormal Psychology*, 85, 167–173.

Silverberg-Shalev, R., Gordon, H. W., Bentin, S., & Aranson, A. (1981). Selective language deterioration in chronic schizophrenia. *Journal of Neurology, Neurosurgery, and Psychiatry,* 44, 547–551.

Spaulding, W. D., Storms, L., Goodrich, V., & Sullivan, M. (1986). Applications of experimental psychopathology in psychiatric rehabilitation. *Schizophrenia Bulletin,* 12, 560–577.

Spring, B. J., Lemon, M., Weinstein, L., & Haskell, A. (1989). Distractibility in schizophrenia: State and trait aspects. *British Journal of Psychiatry,* 155 (suppl. 5), 63–68.

Spring, B. J., & Ravden, L. (in press). Cognitive remediation in schizophrenia: Should we attempt it? *Schizophrenia Bulletin.*

Suddath, R. L., Casanova, M. F., Goldberg, T. E., Daniel, D. G., Kelsoe, J. R., & Weinberger, D. R. (1989). Temporal lobe pathology in schizophrenia: a quantitative magnetic resonance imaging study. *American Journal of Psychiatry,* 146, 464–472.

Tulving, E. (1987). Multiple memory systems and consciousness. *Human Neurobiology,* 6, 67–80.

Wagner, B. R. (1968). The training of attending and abstracting responses in chronic schizophrenics. *Journal of Experimental Research in Personality,* 3, 77–88.

Walker, E. (1981). Attentional and neuromotor functions of schizophrenics, schizoaffectives, and patients with other affective disorders. *Archives of General Psychiatry,* 38, 1355–1358.

Wallace, C. J., & Liberman, R. P. (1985). Social skills training for patients with schizophrenia: A controlled clinical trial. *Psychiatry Research,* 15, 239–247.

Weinberger, D. R., Berman, K. F., & Zec, R. F. (1986) Physiological dysfunction of dorsolateral prefrontal cortex in schizophrenia: I. Regional cerebral blood flow evidence. *Archives of General Psychiatry,* 43, 114–124.

Wishner, J., & Wahl, B. (1974). Dichotic listening in schizophrenia. *Journal of Consulting and Clinical Psychology,* 4, 538–546.

Yu, H. K., & Johnson, J. H. (1979). Imagery in the associative learning of schizophrenics. *Journal of Clinical Psychology,* 35, 265–269.

• 5 •

Cognitive Retraining in a Community Psychiatric Rehabilitation Program

Joel O. Goldberg

Community-based mental health programs are using psychiatric rehabilitation in the form of skills training and support development to facilitate the community adjustment of psychiatrically disabled persons. Like their counterparts in hospital settings, however, community programs have failed to adjust their clinical practices to account for the serious neuropsychological impairments that are so common.

Decades of investigations have chronicled the pervasive impairments in cognitive functioning among individuals with long-term psychiatric disabilities (Heaton, Baade & Johnson, 1978). Up to 75 percent of individuals with schizophrenia may show neuropsychological dysfunction (Taylor & Abrams, 1984). What is perhaps most neglected by community caregivers is the finding that cognitive dysfunctions are evident even after a phase of the client's acute psychosis has subsided (Spaulding, Garbin & Crinean, 1989).

For many years, general clinical practice applied neuropsychological procedures and findings to the narrow assessment question of "schizophrenia versus brain damage" (Malec, 1978). The results, in a sense, were frustratingly unrevealing. When the question is posed in this way, the research literature can only show that individuals with chronic schizophrenia perform as poorly as brain-damaged individuals on neuropsychological tests (Seidman, 1983; Goldstein, 1986). No test pattern has emerged that definitively characterizes only schizophrenic disorders. Recent work has begun to elucidate the neuropathology in schizophrenia by comparing neuropsychological patterns

Partial support of this work was provided by the Ontario Mental Health Foundation. Appreciation is expressed to Dr. Peter E. Cook, Helen Kirkpatrick, Joyce Tryssenaar, and Lori Triano-Antidormi for their contributions and to Roberta Payne for typing the manuscript.

with brain imaging and neurophysiological techniques (Levin, Yurgelum-Todd & and Craft, 1989). What is needed in modern clinical practice, however, is to go beyond the simplistic diagnostic question and make use of what is already known about cognitive impairments to enhance psychiatric rehabilitation strategies.

In this chapter, the impact of neuropsychological dysfunctions on skills training, case management, and community support work is illustrated. Failure to recognize common impairments often results in patients being mislabeled as "lazy," "resistant," "noncompliant" or "passive-aggressive." The second half of this chapter describes how cognitive rehabilitation technologies from work with the head-injured can be adapted to young adults with schizophrenia in a community-based psychiatric rehabilitation program.

Impairments and their Effects on Rehabilitation Practice

1. *Intrusive Ideation (Thought Disorder).* Psychiatric rehabilitation practitioners find that, in community settings, the mere presence of hallucinations, delusions, and bizarre speech ("positive" symptoms of schizophrenia) is often unrelated to the individual's ability to function at work or in everyday living (Brugha et al., 1988). This clinical insight has been supported by longitudinal research that has failed to find a relationship between "positive" symptoms and neuropsychological functioning (Breier et al., 1991). Drugs that reduce thought disorder do not improve intellect (Gold & Hurt, 1990) and they show equivocal effects on other neuropsychological functions (Medalie, Gold & Merriam, 1988), although the side effects of dopamine antagonists and anticholinergic agents may adversely affect motor speed and memory. A crucial implication is that pharmacological interventions that target delusions can be irrelevant to the schizophrenic client's ability to hold a job or manage an apartment.

Community adjustment is determined instead by skills level and adequate support. Some employers or landlords, for example, are naturally more tolerant of unusual symptoms and behavior, or they can be coached in how to react. "Positive" symptoms, though, can be disruptive in social groups, especially among clients who have florid paranoid ideation (Haynes, 1986).

2. *Disorders of Limited Information Capacity.* Information-processing theories of schizophrenia (Knight & Russell, 1978; Callaway & Naghdi, 1982; Gjer-

de, 1983) have speculated that impaired cognitive performance reflects a limit on the capacity of information that can be handled at any single time. New learning or effortful mental operations fail to occur because of high-capacity demands. On the other hand, routine tasks that have become automatic are less strenuous, making minimal capacity demands (Hasher & Zacks, 1979). Some experimental studies consistent with the limited-capacity theory have demonstrated impaired performance by schizophrenic individuals in tasks that require alteration of a previously learned automatic response (Everett, LaPlante & Thomas, 1989). Such findings have important implications for the generalization of skills training interventions.

Some clinicians and family members mistakenly believe that the individual who has limited capacity is being lazy or "resistant." In fact, teachers, for example, should consider that the limited learning capacity of their students is attributable to cognitive overload. As Heinssen and Victor (chap. 9) describe learning a new work skill, even a task as apparently simple as "watering a plant" can have too many information demands until broken down into smaller "chunks." There are many other examples. Restricted information processing capability might be responsible for an individual's inability to deal with more than one issue in a therapy session, or to self-administer complicated medication regimes of several drugs at different times and dosages.

Limited capacity can affect decision making, an area where modern psychiatric rehabilitation practice emphasizes client choice; in the more traditional approach, clinicians tend to be highly directive and to make decisions on behalf of their clients. Yet case management staff report that under the modern approach, individuals are often perseverative in their choices. For example, they identify only very familiar alternatives when facing a choice about their residential, educational, vocational, or social settings, possibly because of the effortful demands in researching new choices. There is a psychiatric rehabilitation technique that works to promote client choice by narrowing options. Cohen et al. (1990) recommend a procedure, called "describing alternative environments," that identifies the three or four best choices from a pool of possibilities, thus helping to brainstorm without overwhelming capacity demands. The idea is that the limited cognitive resources are allocated so that the processing demands do not exceed the available capacity.

3. *Disorders of Attention and Memory.* Clinical descriptions from the time of Emil Kraeplin to the present document the attentional deficits associated

with schizophrenia (Levin, Yurgelun-Todd & Craft, 1988). Recent twin-studies demonstrated that differences in vigilance, memory functioning, and concept formation distinguish the schizophrenic twins from their unaffected monozygotic siblings (Goldberg et al., 1990). Experimental studies have found that attention is impaired on a diverse range of assessment measures because of errors of omission (poor detection). It should be noted, however, that some schizophrenia subtype differences occur. Paranoid schizophrenics can be hypervigilant, making errors of commission by overresponding (Magaro, Johnson & Boring, 1986).

Although attentional dysfunction is often depicted prominently in both the experimental literature and personal accounts, the area is frequently neglected or misunderstood by caregivers and family members. One reason may be that attention and memory problems, while serious, are more subtle than simple lack of alertness. Some schizophrenics have particular difficulty with "deeper" processing of material—for example, by performing less well on recall tasks compared with simple recognition (Larsen & Fromholt, 1976). Goldberg et al. (1989) found that schizophrenic inpatients had difficulty using reminders on a memory task. One suggestion is that the lack of energy (anergia) that clinicians notice in such patients is associated not with laziness but with a specific problem of schizophrenics: they often "forget to remember" (prospective memory). In daily living, "remembering to remember" is crucial to adhering to schedules (as in remembering appointment times). An alternative to the psychodynamic interpretation that blames a client for resistance is a cognitive framework that postulates occasions when prospective memory processes are dysfunctional.

Listed below are some common examples of problems with attention and memory in daily living:

a. Failure to remember an appointment, especially after a shift to a new time. The no-show is often misinterpreted as noncompliance.
b. Failure to shift to a new topic when the conversation flow changes. The mental shift problem is misinterpreted as resistance.
c. Boredom, restlessness, and excessive distractibility in groups or activities that demand sustained attention for lengthy periods. The poor vigilance is misinterpreted as laziness or lack of interest.
d. Failure to attend to personal hygiene without prompting, even when knowledgeable about self-care. Skills teaching is often redun-

dant in this case, since what is needed is training to initiate performance or supportive reminder cues.

e. Becoming sharply focused on a particular detail to the extent of losing sight of the broader picture, characteristic especially of those who are suspicious.

4. *Disorders of Problem Solving.* The ability to plan and then initiate a course of purposeful action, to integrate behavior into meaningful activity, and to develop and maintain a level of aroused interest are cognitive processes termed executive functions (Levin et al., 1989). They are thought to be mediated by frontal lobe systems. In fact, known frontal lobe dysfunction can produce delusions very similar to the symptoms and clinical picture of paranoid schizophrenia, suggesting a common defect in frontal lobe functioning (Benson & Stuss, 1990). Further supporting this line of thinking, imaging studies show an association between poor categorization skills on the Wisconsin Card Sort Test and prefrontal cortex dysfunction (Weinberger, Berman & Zec, 1986).

Individuals with schizophrenia can show striking error patterns on problem-solving tests. When they try to solve problems that require a shift from a previously successful strategy, schizophrenics tend to perseverate (Kolb & Whishaw, 1983); that is, they keep repeating the original strategy even though it no longer works (Goldberg et al., 1987).

In the verbal area, disordered language can be associated with unusually concrete expressions of incoherent ideas, as shown by studies that examine the ability to formulate stories (Allen, 1984). Such literal thinking may reflect difficulties in arranging and organizing meaningful material into ideas.

Finally, individuals may fail to develop and exercise the drive necessary to solve problems (Frith & Done, 1988). Rather than misattributing such problems to a character trait—poor motivation—caregivers should consider that there may be dysfunctions in the executive system responsible for initiating the action. Rehabilitation training can go astray by teaching basic skills that are already known when the actual impairment is in the planning, drive, and integration functions that prompt the utilization of the skills.

CASE 1

Client G.A. is a 27-year-old male with an 8-year history of schizophrenia and several long hospitalizations. He receives social assistance and lives in a boarding home. Crisis phone calls are frequent when his money runs out, precipitating demands for readmission. In budget training sessions, it has been found that he shows excellent calculation ability. For example, he knows the price of cigarette packages and can easily make change. Instead, he has impairment at the executive systems level, which prevents him from dividing his income allowance into segments that will last a whole month.

The central feature of psychiatric rehabilitation (Anthony, Cohen & Farkas, 1990) is overall goal-directed planning, not just skills training and support development. When a rehabilitation plan has been established, distinctions are made between lack of skills (which would require the intervention of skills teaching) and limited use of skills (which might require the development of supports or skills programming). For example, a client may be capable of performing household chores but fails to do them without prompting. Such "defect in the initiation of spontaneous action" can be a component of the neuropsychology of schizophrenia, according to Frith & Done (1988).

Approaches to Cognitive Rehabilitation

To illustrate the three main approaches to cognitive rehabilitation, consider a youngster with a visual impairment who has been mislabeled lazy or resistant in the classroom by the teacher. To address the problem, three avenues of intervention can be identified. The "adjustment to loss" approach would move the shortsighted youngster from the rear to the front of the classroom, where the blackboard could be seen. The "strategy-building" or coping approach would mitigate the effects of the visual problem through eyeglasses. The "train the brain," or retraining, approach would exercise a weak eye by covering the stronger eye with a patch until optimal function has been restored. These three approaches, adjustment, coping, and retraining, are convenient ways of categorizing the levels at which neuropsychological principles have been applied to rehabilitation interventions.

1. *Adjustment to Loss.* In the adjustment approach, a comprehensive neuropsychological assessment specifies adaptive strengths and weaknesses relevant to skills of everyday living. Unlike older procedures aimed at predicting locus of lesions, or diagnosing pathology, a modern evaluation examines functions as a means of planning rehabilitation efforts. Such individual descriptions of patterns of preserved and impaired abilities have determined re-

habilitation plans in treating head injuries for the past decade (Goldstein & Ruthven, 1983), but they are only beginning to be used in this manner in psychiatric rehabilitation (Yozawitz, 1986).

The major rehabilitative focus is adjusting plans in the living, learning, work, and social areas to capitalize on strengths and to minimize weakness.

> CASE 2
>
> Client D.S. was struggling in his part-time job despite good eye-hand coordination skills that made carrying out his actual duties quite easy. Careful examination of the implicit job requirements showed that his supervisor was a talkative person who conversed frequently with the employees. D.S. did not have the verbal or social abilities to manage the conversational skills demanded in this job setting. Plans were adjusted to a quieter setting with a friendly but less verbal supervisor.

Erickson (1988; Erickson & Burton, 1986) uses a neuropsychological test protocol to screen a variety of cognitive skills as the basis for adjusting rehabilitation plans (Erickson & Burton, 1986). Just as the shortsighted student was seated near the blackboard, so the perseverative patient is engaged in highly structured regular routine with few changes. Individuals with persistence problems are scheduled for shorter but more frequent sessions. In a similar vein, Liberman, Nuechterlein & Wallace (1982) recommend uncluttered training settings, devoid of distractions for patients with attention problems.

A key challenge for rehabilitation-oriented neuropsychologists is finding areas of strength in individuals who have significant disability. Dalby & Williams (1986) have suggested that, not unlike organic dementias, schizophrenia spectrum disorders may coexist with preserved reading and spelling ability. Other studies (Feitel & Sano, 1983) have found that more than half of young adult chronic patients are functionally illiterate. Since literacy is so important to community adjustment, achievement skills testing should investigate whether illiteracy is hampering success in training programs.

2. *Strategy-Building*. In the strategy-building approach, coping devices or prostheses assist in carrying out functions. Analogous to eyeglasses that mitigate the effects of visual problems, a variety of compensatory strategies and technologies are being used in psychiatric rehabilitation.

In community housing, some apartment projects have insulated flooring to provide sound barriers against pacing, which otherwise might result in tenant complaints and ejection by landlords. Bathrooms are posted with reminder notices for hygiene routines, and work settings have charts showing the correct order of skill sequences (cf. Heinssen in chap. 9 of this volume).

Attention and memory problems can be partially relieved through coping devices such as medication dosettes, boxes with small compartments designed to hold pills, labeled for each time period of the day and each day of the week. Clients can use dosettes to aid self-administration of medication and thereby increase independent functioning. Weekly schedules and diaries are common aids for memory troubles (Sohlberg & Mateer, 1989).

A more comprehensive approach has been described for coping with disorders of problem solving. Zec and Meisler (1986) construct decks of job cards that clients can use to organize and monitor the correct order of their task behaviors. This "executive board system" has been hypothesized to compensate for both impaired ability to shift set and defective initiative through explicit information (recorded on cue cards) about the timing and sequencing of tasks. Reinforcing feedback is provided by transferring the completed job card into the appropriate card pocket.

Survey studies and personal accounts can provide important information about the kinds of coping methods that individuals with schizophrenia have found to compensate for disordered cognition in everyday life. Carr (1988) asked 200 individuals with schizophrenia who were living in the community to report on their coping strategies. Almost half said they employed distraction techniques, generally listening to music. One increasingly common device is a compact, wearable radio with headset (known as a Walkman), which may serve the purpose of shifting attention from internal to external experiences. There is a report of the successful use of an earplug to minimize attention to auditory hallucinations (Done, Frith & Owens, 1986). Hatfield's (1989) brief review of first-person accounts showed that cognitive confusion and attentional deficits are frequently reported. The most common "prosthesis," however, appears to be social support. Ironically, occasional reliance on a helpful person to assist in solving problems can be pejoratively labeled as "dependency" in psychiatry, while the aid of an attendant to cope with a physical handicap is seen as supportive in rehabilitation.

3. *Train the Brain.* The most controversial approach for individuals with schizophrenia is the application of the cognitive retraining technology used with the head-injured. A basic premise of retraining is that remediation oc-

curs through exercise of neuronal circuits by imposing information processing demands. Cognitive skills are trained or recovered through practice at tasks. Benedict (1989) reviewed the outcome literature on cognitive remediation of people with head injuries. An important finding is that attention training is essential since other brain systems depend on attention for effective cognitive processing (Gummow, Miller & Dustman, 1983). It is unclear at this point whether the cognitive disorders associated with schizophrenia can be retrained.

Promising cognitive training work with psychiatric populations has been reported, but shortcomings limit the utility of the findings. Diamant (1986) published a brief descriptive paper on the future of microcomputer training with psychiatric patients, but there were no empirical analyses. Benedict and Harris (1989) note in a brief report that microcomputer training can improve simple reaction times, but they recommend further work to determine whether attention training can enhance performance of other tasks. Olbrich and Mussgay (1990) describe a failure to find improvements after cognitive retraining with schizophrenic individuals. However, in this European study the subjects were acutely psychotic inpatients and the length of training was only three weeks. Thus, the results cannot be generalized to stabilized chronic patients undergoing long-term rehabilitation.

In the area of problem solving, Bellack et al. (1990) found that poor card sorting could be alleviated with brief training. Their technique of training for learning the Wisconsin Card Sort produced improved retest performance but clearly confounded independent and dependent measures. The question remains whether the training effects could generalize to other categorization tasks. An additional problem with previous work, especially microcomputer training, is that the exercises involve predominantly the visual modality. Although individuals with schizophrenia can show visual attention problems, there is also great need to work with auditory and listening skills, since natural environments demand such capability.

Pilot Studies: Attention Training in Schizophrenia

Given the growing recognition of the relative importance of attention impairments in schizophrenia (e.g., Saykin et al., 1991), we reviewed the literature on cognitive interventions to identify retraining technology that targets attention problems.

Early methods to retrain attention in a schizophrenic were reported by Adams et al. (1981). The intervention was quite brief (nine sessions), the rehabilitation technology used was in its infancy (repeated practice, followed by tasks such as Digit Span as dependent measures). Another limitation of this research was that the treatment was combined with cognitive-behavioral procedures, and the impact of the attention training thus could not be isolated (Magaro, Johnson & Boring 1986).

In the head injury literature, there have been a number of published case reports of successful attention retraining (Benedict 1989). The most promising technology that has emerged is the theory-based Attention Process Training (APT), designed by Sohlberg and Mateer (1987). APT is a major advance because the exercises are diverse (both auditory and visual) and progress through graduated stages of difficulty and increasing complexity of information-processing tasks (see table 5.1). Unlike studies that confound outcome measures with the treatment tasks, APT is a six-month program that uses independent measures to show generalized improvements on attention tests beyond the training exercises.

We have begun a series of single case studies to determine whether APT can be used to train attentional problems found in schizophrenia.

CASE 3

Client M.G. is a 29-year-old male outpatient with a 10-year prior history of paranoid ideas and vague, digressive speech. He has had three psychiatric admissions and was being treated with Fluanxol, Haldol, and Clonazepam. His pretraining MMPI confirmed the clinical diagnosis of schizophrenia, with a schizophrenia scale peak over 90 and the only other elevations on D and Hs for an 8*21 psychotic codetype. Intelligence was impaired (Verbal IQ = 71, Performance IQ = 62, Full Scale IQ = 65) with even worse attention functioning (WMS – MQ = 58). On the Halstead-Reitan indices, he showed severe impairment (global impairment index = 1.0).

M.G. clearly benefited from five months of training, showing improvements in his recall of a drawing of the Rey Figure (see figs. 5.1 and 5.2). According to functional reports, his boarding home operator stated that he does not have to be reminded to show up for meals. The trainer found he can better sustain conversations. His case manager found it no longer necessary to provide a written schedule of his weekly

Table 5.1: Steps in Attention Process Training and Associated Impairments

1. Focused attention (intact for psychiatrically disabled)
   Impairment: Lacks alertness
   Exercises: Practice response to stimuli

2. Sustained attention
   Impairment: Lacks mental control
   Performance fluctuates
   Focus is too brief
   Exercises: Practice response maintenance

3. Selective attention
   Impairment: Easily distracted
   Exercises: Practice response with distractors

4. Alternating attention
   Impairment: Problems shifting set
   Exercise: Practice mental flexibility

5. Divided attention
   Impairment: Can do only one thing at a time
   Exercise: Practice multiple responses

routine, an essential coping aid that compensated for his recall problems.

The initial results encouraged a more formal case study evaluation, which was conducted at our community-based program as part of a master's thesis project (Tryssenaar 1990). Findings from her study replicated and extended the success of APT with a second client, a 26-year-old male diagnosed with schizoaffective disorder.

Results of this case study (see fig. 5.3) showed improved attention on measures that were not part of the practicing, specifically the Rey Figure (visual recall) and Paced Auditory Serial Addition Test (PASAT; auditory attention). A dramatic change was also found on his Wechsler Memory Scale: the memory quotient rose from the low-average pretraining level (WMS-MQ = 86) to an above-average posttraining score (WMS-MQ = 112). The client's improvements generalized to daily functioning, according to family members, the employer, the clinician, and self-reports. There were no changes on a control task measure of spatial processing, which replicates the pattern of results found by Sohlberg and Mateer (1987) for head-injured clients.

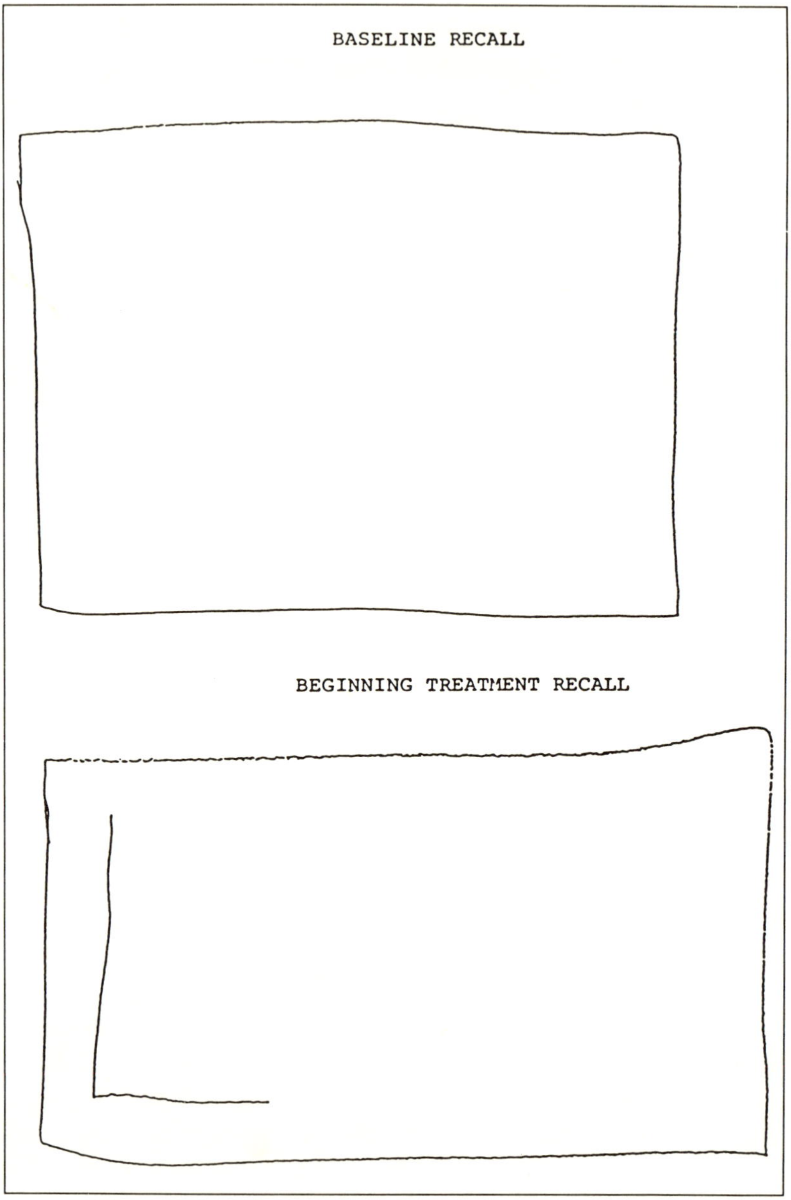

Figure 5.1: Baseline Rey Figure recall (Client M.G.)

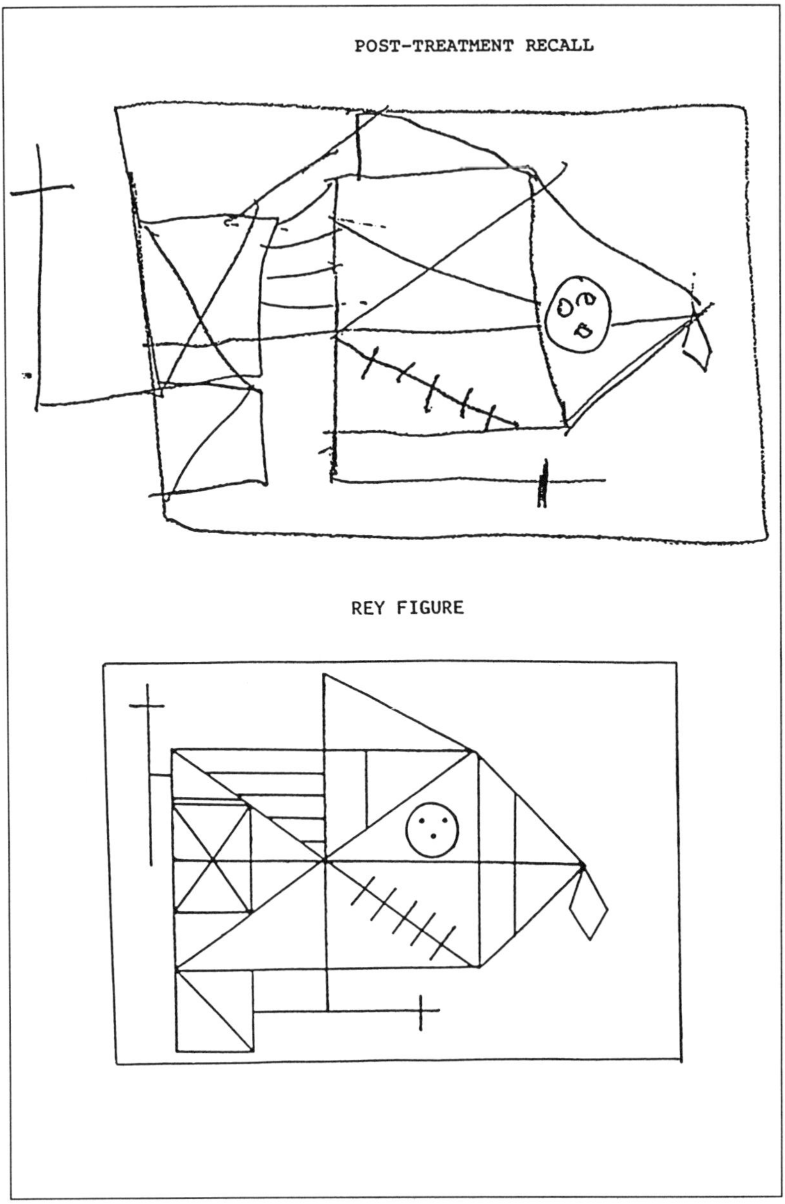

Figure 5.2: Outcome Rey Figure recall (Client M.G.)

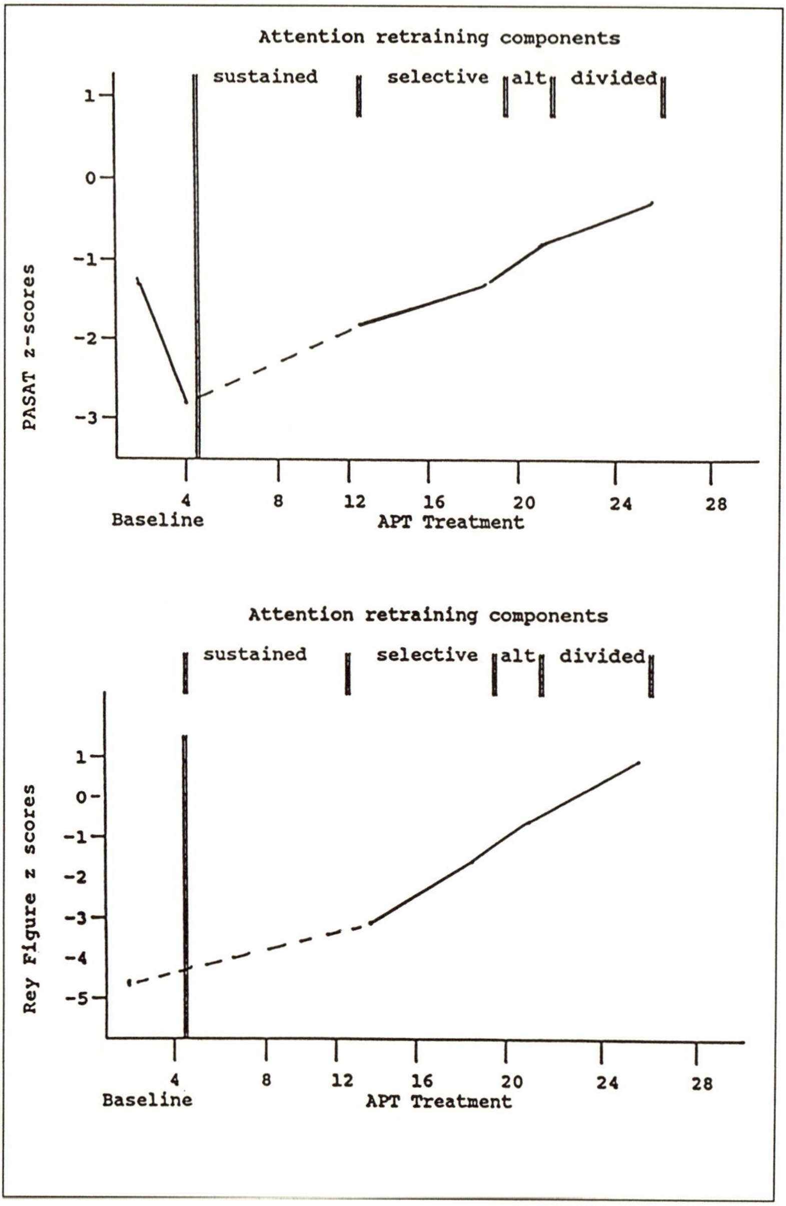

Figure 5.3: Results of APT *cognitive training on attention measures (Client L. G.)*

Conclusion

The majority of clients who attend community-based psychiatric rehabilitation programs have significant cognitive impairments. Often unrecognized, problems such as poor attention and dysfunctional planning skills are misinterpreted as laziness or resistance or are given various psychodynamic interpretations. Mental health professionals may find it helpful to identify the ways in which cognitive abnormalities actually disrupt daily living, learning, work, and social activities. The emerging field of cognitive rehabilitation provides three avenues for intervening: adjustment to loss, strategy-building, and retraining.

Looking to the future of cognitive rehabilitation, there will be a critical need for the technological development and elaboration of strategies in these three areas if intervention work is to proceed effectively.

In the adjustment-to-loss approach, a crucial step is making neuropsychological assessments relevant to daily functioning. This represents a shift from the purely diagnostic approach ("find the organicity") of past decades. Assessment reports should integrate the neuropsychological formulations into functional suggestions and recommendations that health care professionals can use in designing adjustment plans. Neuropsychological evaluations may eventually provide a bridge between findings from advanced brain-imaging techniques and impaired cognitive skills.

The strategy-building approach depends on creative coping techniques, changes in environments, and "prosthetic" devices. Surveys of mental health consumers reveal that they have discovered cognitive coping strategies beyond taking pills. There is an urgent need to develop, evaluate, and systematize supportive resources, including coping devices, that can assist those with cognitive disabilities in adjusting most independently.

Use of the retraining approach with psychiatric disorders is still in its infancy. Like the findings with the head-injured, there are promising results in retraining attention, based on a small number of case studies. Much more research needs to be done in substantiating preliminary pilot work with controlled outcome studies, so that claims for success are supported by efficacy data. Significant advances in inventing retraining technology are more likely to come from theory-based methods, such as APT, rather than atheoretical approaches that offer simple exposure to practice exercises.

References

Adams, H. E., Malatesta, V., Brantley, P. J., & Turkat, I. D. (1981). Modification of cognitive processes: A case study in schizophrenia. *Journal of Clinical and Consulting Psychology*, 49, 460–464.

Allen, H. A. (1984). Positive and negative symptoms and the thematic organization of schizophrenic speech. *British Journal of Psychiatry*, 144, 611–617.

Anthony, W., Cohen, M., & Farkas, M. (1990). *Psychiatric rehabilitation*. Boston: Boston University, Center for Psychiatric Rehabilitation.

Bellack, A. S., Mueser, K. T., Morrison, R. L., et al. (1990). Remediation of cognitive deficits in schizophrenia. *American Journal of Psychiatry*, 147, 1650–1655.

Benedict, R. H. B. (1989). The effectiveness of cognitive remediation strategies for victims of traumatic head-injury: A review of the literature. *Clinical Psychology Review*, 9, 605–626.

Benedict, R. H. B., & Harris, A. E. (1989). Remediation of attention deficits in chronic schizophrenic patients: A preliminary study. *British Journal of Clinical Psychology*, 28, 187–188.

Benson, D. F., & Stuss, D. T. (1990). Frontal lobe influences on delusions: A clinical perspective. *Schizophrenia Bulletin*, 16, 403–412.

Brier, A., Schreiber J. L., Dyer, J., & Pickar, D. (1991). NIMH longitudinal study of chronic schizophrenia. *Archives of General Psychiatry*, 48, 239–246.

Brugha, T. S., Wing, J. K., Brewin, C. R., et al. (1988). The problems of people in long-term psychiatric day care. *Psychological Medicine*, 18, 443–456.

Callaway, E., & Naghdi, M. A. (1982). An information processing model for schizophrenia. *Archives of General Psychiatry*, 39, 339–347.

Carr, V. (1988). Patients' techniques for coping with schizophrenia: An exploratory study. *British Journal of Medical Psychology*, 61, 339–352.

Cohen, M. R., Farkas, M. D., Cohen B. F., & Unger, K. V. (1990). *Psychiatric rehabilitation technology: Setting an overall rehabilitation goal (Trainer package)*. Boston: Boston University, Center for Psychiatric Rehabilitation.

Dalby, J. T., & Williams, R. (1986). Preserved reading and spelling ability in psychotic disorders. *Psychological Medicine*, 16, 171–175.

Diamant, J. J. (1986). Specific features of cognitive rehabilitation of psychiatric patients. *Cognitive Rehabilitation*, 4, 12–26.

Done, D. J., Frith, C. D., & Owens, D. C. (1986). Reducing persistent auditory hallucinations by wearing an ear plug. *British Journal of Clinical Psychology*, 25, 151–152.

Erickson, R. C. (1988). Neuropsychological assessment and the rehabilitation of persons with severe psychiatric disabilities. *Rehabilitation Psychology*, 33, 15–24.

Erickson, R. C., & Burton, M. A. (1986). Working with psychiatric patients with cognitive deficits. *Cognitive Rehabilitation*, 4, 26–31.

Everett, J., Laplante, L., & Thomas, J. (1989). The selective attention deficit in schizophrenia: Limited resources or cognitive fatigue? *Journal of Nervous and Mental Disease,* 177, 735–738.

Feitel, B., & Sano, M. (1983). Intellectual assessment of young adult chronic patients. *Hospital and Community Psychiatry,* 34, 1153–1155.

Frith, C. D., & Done, D. J. (1988). Towards a neuropsychology of schizophrenia. *British Journal of Psychiatry,* 153, 437–443.

Gjerde, P. F. (1983). Attention capacity dysfunction and arousal in schizophrenia. *Psychological Bulletin,* 93, 57–72.

Gold, J. M., & Hurt, S. W. (1990). The effects of haloperidol on thought disorder and IQ in schizophrenia. *Journal of Personality Assessment,* 54, 390–400.

Goldberg, T. E., Ragland, J. D., Fuller-Torrey, E., et al. (1990). Neuropsychological assessment of monozygotic twins discordant for schizophrenia. *Archives of General Psychiatry,* 47, 1066–1072.

Goldberg, T. E., Weinberger, D. R., Berman, K. F., et al. (1987). Further evidence for dementia of the prefrontal type in schizophrenia? A controlled study of teaching the Wisconsin Card Sort Test. *Archives of General Psychiatry,* 44, 1008–1014.

Goldberg, T. E., Weinberger, D. R., Pliskin, N. H., Berman, K. F., & Podd, M. H. (1989). Recall memory deficit in schizophrenia: a possible manifestation of prefrontal dysfunction. *Schizophrenia Research,* 2, 251–257.

Goldstein, G. (1986). The neuropsychology of schizophrenia. In I. Grant and K. M. Adams, (Eds.), *Neuropsychological assessment of neuropsychiatric disorders.* New York: Oxford Press.

Goldstein, G., & Ruthven, L. (1983). Neuropsychological testing as a means of planning rehabilitation programs. In G. Goldstein and L. Ruthven (Eds.), *Rehabilitation of the brain-damaged adult.* New York: Plenum Press.

Gummow, L., Miller, P., & Dustman, R. (1983). Attention and brain injury: A case for cognitive rehabilitation of attentional deficits. *Clinical Psychology Review,* 3, 255–274.

Hasher, L., & Zacks, R. T. (1979). Automatic and effortful processes in memory. *Journal of Experimental Psychology (General),* 108, 356–388.

Hatfield, A. (1989). Patients' accounts of stress and coping in schizophrenia. *Hospital and Community Psychiatry,* 40, 1141–1145.

Haynes, S. N. (1986). A behavioral model of paranoid behaviors. *Behavior Therapy,* 17, 266–287.

Heaton, R. K., Baede, L. E., & Johnson, K. L. (1978). Neuropsychological test results associated with psychiatric disorders in adults. *Psychological Bulletin,* 85, 141–162.

Knight, R. G., & Russell, P. N. (1978). Global capacity reduction and schizophrenia. *British Journal of Social and Clinical Psychology,* 17, 275–280.

Kolb, B., & Whishaw, I. Q. (1983). Performance of schizophrenic patients on tests sensitive to left or right frontal, temporal or parietal function in neurological patients. *Journal of Nervous and Mental Disease,* 171, 435–443.

Larsen, S. F., & Fromholt, P. (1976). Mnemonic organization and free recall in schizophrenia. *Journal of Abnormal Psychology,* 85, 61–65.

Levin, S., Yurgelin-Todd, D., & Craft, S. (1989). Contributions of clinical neuropsychology to the study of schizophrenia. *Journal of Abnormal Psychology,* 98, 341–356.

Liberman, R. P., Neuchterlein, K., & Wallace, D. (1982). Social skills training and the nature of schizophrenia. In J. Curran and P. Monti (Eds.), *Social skills training: A practical handbook for assessment and treatment.* New York: Guilford Press.

Magaro, P. A., Johnson, M. H., & Boring, R. (1986). Information processing approaches to the treatment of schizophrenia. In R. E. Ingram (Ed.), *Information processing approaches to clinical psychology.* New York: Academic Press.

Malec, J. (1978). Neuropsychological assessment of schizophrenia versus brain damage: A review. *Journal of Nervous and Mental Disease,* 166, 507–516.

Medalie, A., Gold, J., & Merriam, A. (1988). The effects of neuroleptics on neuropsychological test results of schizophrenics. *Archives of Clinical Neuropsychology,* 3, 249–271.

Olbrich, R., & Mussgay, L. (1990). Reduction of schizophrenic deficits by cognitive training: An evaluative study. *European Archives of Psychiatry and Neurological Sciences,* 239, 366–369.

Saykin, A. J., Gur, R. C., Gur, R. E., et al. (1991). Neuropsychological function in schizophrenia: Selective impairment in memory and learning. *Archives of General Psychiatry,* 48, 618–624.

Seidman, L. J. (1983). Schizophrenia and brain dysfunction: An integration of recent neurodiagnostic findings. *Psychological Bulletin,* 94, 195–238.

Sohlberg, M., & Mateer, C. M. (1987). Effectiveness of an attention training program. *Journal of Clinical and Experimental Neuropsychology,* 9(2), 117–130.

Sohlberg, M. M., & Mateer, C. A. (1989). Training use of compensatory memory books: A three-stage behavioral approach. *Journal of Clinical and Experimental Neuropsychology,* 11, 871–891.

Spaulding, W., Garbin, C. P., & Crinean, W. J. (1989). The logical and psychometric prerequisites for cognitive therapy of schizophrenia. *British Journal of Psychiatry,* 155 (suppl. 5), 69–73.

Taylor, M. A., & Abrams, R. (1984). Cognitive impairment in schizophrenia. *American Journal of Psychiatry,* 141, 196–201.

Tryssenaar, J. (1990). The efficacy of cognitive retraining of attention deficits for a client who has schizophrenia. Unpublished master's thesis, Brock University, St. Catharines, Ont., Canada.

Weinberger, D. R., Berman, K. F., & Zec, R. F. (1986). Physiologic dysfunction of dorsolateral prefrontal cortex in schizophrenia. *Archives of General Psychiatry,* 43, 114–124.

Yozawitz, A. (1986). Applied neuropsychology in a psychiatric center. In J. Gant & K. Adams (Eds.) *Neuropsychological assessment of neuropsychiatric disorders.* New York: Oxford Press.

Zec, R. F., & Meisler, N. (1986). Executive Board System (EBS): A self-help approach to cognitive-behavior rehabilitation. Paper presented at the International Association of Psychosocial Rehabilitation Services meetings, Cleveland, Ohio.

•6•

Reframing Rehabilitation: Putting Skill Acquisition and the Mental Health System into Proper Perspective

Susan B. Fine

This chapter addresses the problems of schizophrenia within a systems context: the biopsychosocial system that influences the individual's capacities to fulfill life roles and responsibilities, and the mental health system that influences access to meaningful and effective treatment resources. Emphasis is placed on the importance of perspective—in understanding the tenacious deficit behaviors of schizophrenia and in developing more responsive treatment strategies and service systems that support function in the chronically mentally ill. First, an overview of current neurobehavioral thinking about the interactive nature of impaired functioning provides the foundation for a discussion of a multicontextual rehabilitation strategy, Task Oriented Learning Therapy (TOLT). TOLT organizes cognitive and social skills acquisition interventions in a graded, individualized manner that supports generalization to community living. The process of strategy development and the position of rehabilitation in the larger system of mental health services is also discussed within the context of current initiatives in New York State.

Issues in Rehabilitation: Failures and Fortitude

While there are some who proclaim psychiatric rehabilitation to be a "bold new approach," concerns for patients' functional capacities have a long, if often lonely, history. A historical look at psychiatric and physical rehabilitation provides a fascinating social-political-economic picture of an idea whose time has come and gone—again, and again, and again (Anthony & Liberman, 1986; Christianson, 1991; Fine, 1980; Gritzer & Arluke, 1985; Liberman,

1988; Meyer, 1922). If anything were to be described as bold or new, it would be (1) the acknowledgement that patients are more than their illness, and (2) sustained interdisciplinary commitment to the complex biopsychosocial elements of chronic mental illness (Fine, 1980).

Happily, there has been progress. The persistent efforts of practitioners, basic scientists, patients, families, and other advocates have heightened the visibility of psychiatric rehabilitation; enriched our understanding of the relationships among disease, disability, discrimination, and adaptation; initiated model treatment programs; produced more trained rehabilitation specialists; and generated research activities.

However, these efforts are occurring during a prolonged period of upheaval within all sectors of the health care system. Drastic fiscal constraints, shorter lengths of stay, inadequate aftercare programs, interdisciplinary competition for shrinking resources, and consumer and third-party payer demands for measurable and meaningful outcomes have sorely challenged the most resilient organizations and clinicians. Rehabilitation, along with other specialties, is being put to very rigorous tests, and justifiably so. For, in spite of recent gains, the art and science of psychiatric rehabilitation has not fully fulfilled its promise.

WHY DOESN'T REHABILITATION WORK BETTER

The difficulties we experience in effecting change in the functional behaviors of many schizophrenic individuals are multidetermined and cannot simply be ascribed to the complex, tenacious nature of the illness itself. Rehabilitation technology and the mental health system must accept a significant share of responsibility. There are not enough programs and skilled practitioners available for those in need of functionally oriented services. Acute care settings, which provide the largest but briefest share of psychiatric services, tend to follow a crisis-intervention model, with little attention to the functional dimensions and sequelae of the disease. Time contraints and a biomedical disease orientation often misguidedly relegate daily living skills and community adaptation to the postdischarge phase alone. Since too few rehabilitation resources are available in the community, survival is a difficult and lonely process for those without necessary skills and access to treatment and support services. Many patients relapse and require rehospitalization.

There are also problems with the quality and appropriateness of aftercare services that are available. Many programs fail to promote continuity of care or to provide realistic, individualized interventions that acknowledge and accommodate underlying impairments and fluctuations in symptoms and functioning. Also, in the absence of sufficient research data supporting programmatic claims, limited resources have not always been directed to the most promising interventions.

Even without hard data, high recidivism and relapse among those completing rehabilitation programs send a strong negative message. There continues to be a disparity between the needs of consumers and the treatment methods in common use. In a compelling discussion of so-called schizophrenic resistance to social and vocational rehabilitation, Hogarty (1985) points to the lack of fit between patients' capacities and deficits, the field's understanding of these deficits, and the methods and goals of treatment. He cites "premature expectations or prescriptions of therapeutic tasks that require adaptive efficiency, cognitive integration and insight beyond patient capability" (p. 4) as a major provocation of outcome failures and symptom exacerabation. Failures are particularly commonplace among patients with persistent deficit symptoms.

The work described in this chapter (conducted in the Department of Psychiatry, New York Hospital–Cornell University Medical Center) has found its inspiration in these very failures, in patients' painful sense of having little control over themselves and their environment, and in the lack of control that staff experience in dealing with unremitting symptoms and poor treatment outcomes. Although these two types of failure are reason enough to pursue new, more effective strategies, a third element, emerging neuroscientific evidence linking deficit symptoms with cerebral defects, has added exciting substance to efforts to overcome the adversity of persistent functional impairments. These issues provide a context for reexamining the reasoning behind many contemporary treatment efforts and for reframing the rehabilitation process.

The Phenomenology of Schizophrenia and the Failure to Function

For many individuals afflicted with the debilitating symptoms of schizophrenia, the most rudimentary tasks of daily living in unsympathetic environments present overwhelming challenges. The experience is best conveyed by those who struggle with the disease's impact on personal identity, sense of purpose, social relationships, and future orientation. In a personal account, McGrath (1982) captures the dilemma by comparing herself to "the rear tire of a bicycle, not trusted enough to be the front tire, expected to go round and round in one narrow rut, never going very far, ignored except when I break down . . . put into a garage, sometimes for months, where I forget my function and . . . become afraid to function and all functions seem useless" (p. 21).

POSITIVE AND NEGATIVE SYMPTOMS

Since there is little to recommend schizophrenia, it may appear strange to the uninitiated, and certainly to those who struggle with the disease, to speak of its "positive" and "negative" symptoms. Nonetheless, clinicians and neuroscientists make that important distinction, for schizophrenia is not all of one piece. The construct of negative/positive symptom syndromes establishes important distinctions between florid symptoms and residual deficit behaviors that impede social and personal function (Andreason, 1982a, 1982b, 1985; Carpenter et al., 1973).

Positive symptoms are characterized by prominent delusions, hallucinations, a formal thought disorder, and bizarre behavior. These florid manifestations are viewed as distortions of normal function. Patients with only these symptoms generally reflect better premorbid adjustment and better overall function, and they show no evidence of cerebral atrophy when compared to those with negative symptoms (Andreason, 1982b). In contrast, the negative symptom cluster is characterized by a loss of normal function: affective flattening, poverty of speech, apathy, social withdrawal, impaired social judgment, inability to sustain attention and carry tasks to completion, and difficulties in changing mental sets and solving problems. These patients have had poor premorbid adjustment, lower overall levels of function, impaired cognition, often some history of previous brain injury, and cerebral atrophy (Andreason, 1982b). These residual deficits influence self-care, relationships, work, leisure-time pursuits, overall community adjustment, the frequency of relapse and rehospitalization, and capacities to engage in and benefit from treatment and rehabilitation. These syndromes may occur alone or in combination.

Care must be taken not to oversimplify or overapply the negative symptom construct, since there are other conditions, such as medication side effects, depression, and long-term exposure to isolation and unstimulating environments, that elicit similar behaviors. These secondary effects, usually amenable to changes in medication and milieu, should not be taken for, or treated as, primary deficit symptoms (Carpenter et al., 1985; Carpenter, 1991).

THE COGNITIVE CORE

The behaviors identified in Andreason's Scale for the Assessment of Negative Symptoms (1983) reflect key areas of attentional and cognitive deficits known to impede functional performance. They include difficulty in sustaining forcused attention, distractibility, slowness in initial processing of information in sensory memory, impaired detection of relevant stimuli embedded in irrelevant noise, and inefficient active organization of information in short-term memory (Koh, 1978; McGhie et al., 1965; Rappaport et al., 1972;-Saccuzzo et al., 1974; Wolberg & Kornetsky, 1973). These components of cognition are extremely important for fulfilling the tasks and interpersonal demands of daily living. They are the means by which we acquire and process information, learn, generalize one experience to others, and make adaptations to environmental demands (Abreu & Toglia, 1987).

The influence of underlying cognitive deficits on performance emerges in the treatment environment as well. Clinicians routinely report patients' difficulties with concentration, memory, self-monitoring, and generalization from clinic to community, although the status of these skills is often ignored in selecting treatment tasks requiring higher levels of cognitive competency than a given patient possesses. For example, we attempt to enhance social skills through practice and reinforcement with role playing in group settings—in spite of of the fact that these modalities are interpersonally and cognitively demanding and are rich in arousal potential. In effect, we fail to consider the fact that many social skills deficits are, in part, the manifestation of basic underlying cognitive deficits (Toglia & Golisz, 1990). We need to remind ourselves that attention deficits produce tendencies to drift off the topic of conversation and that they decrease awareness of the nonverbal and verbal reactions of others. Poor memory causes difficulties in keeping track of conversations, and rigidity of thought processes curtails abilities to see other points of view and to come up with alternatives to social problems. Role playing involves taking the perspective of others in interpersonal situations; like the social skills one wishes to develop, it requires participants to deal with more than one perspective at a time. The absence of a well-synchronized cognitive infrastructure makes the learning and generalization of these skills in stimulus-rich group settings difficult and unpredictable at best. At worst, such overload experiences may serve as powerful stressors that trigger the very symptoms we wish to contain.

Brenner (1987) suggests that an inadequate understanding of "the intermediate processes between pre-existing vulnerability characteristics and manifest behavior disorders" (p. 138) generates nonspecific and, therefore, ineffective treatment interventions. Task performance, with or without manifest interpersonal elements, makes demands on and requires the integration of major elements of information processing identified by Luria (1980) as alertness and basic attentional skills; discrimination of information from environment; and internal planning, decision making, and problem solving. Tasks that are not routine, that require thinking, judging, planning, and assimilating new and rapidly changing information—or that involve risk—place increased demands on each of these functions (Vezzetti, 1989). In individuals whose cognitive "hardware" is faulty to begin with, the system's capacity to respond is obviously compromised.

The Contributions of Neuroscience

Although the presumption of a neurobiological dimension to schizophrenia is a long-standing one, neuroscientists have only recently been able to produce respectable data linking physiological abnormalities of the brain to the disease. Anomalies in ventricular size and limbic structures (Owens et al., 1985; Meltzer, 1987), metabolic anomalies in the frontal cortex (Weinberger et al., 1986), left hemisphere cognitive dysfunction (Gazzaniga, 1988), and variations in neurochemical activites (Meltzer & Sahl, 1976) are of particular relevance. Current research efforts emphasize the interaction of various brain systems at many levels, rather than a single focal flaw (NIMH, 1988). These findings provide a challenging framework for understanding the cognitive impairments and aberrant social behaviors associated with schizophrenia. The reader is referred to this chapter's bibliography and to the other chapters in this volume to pursue these themes in greater detail. There are, however, several issues that merit some elaboration here.

DOPAMINE, EYE TRACKING, AND SCHIZOPHRENIA

Abnormalities in dopamine production, particularly in the limbic system, have been linked with negative and positive symptom syndromes and with difficulties in integrating environmental data and preparing adequate responses from cortical areas (Meltzer & Stahl, 1976). The relationships among dopamine production, irregularities of motor activity, and performance capacities have been explored in research relating eye-tracking dysfunction and schizophrenic "thought slippage" (Holtzman, 1985). The prevalence of eye-movement disorders (both smooth pursuit and saccadic movements) among schizophrenics and their first-degree relatives is of some importance, since these movements influence accurate perception and cognitive centering (Leigh & Zee, 1983). Although relationships among visual motor perception, cognition, and daily performance are familiar issues for occupational therapists in physical rehabilitation (Abreu & Toglia, 1987), mental health specialists of all persuasions have not adequately considered these factors in their work with this population. Gibson's (1986) "theory of affordances," an action-in-the-environment model in which sensory information is given meaning through experience in the real world, provides a useful frame of reference for dealing with perceptual and cognitive problems in schizophrenia.

GENDER ISSUES

The preponderance of chronically ill males with poor rehabilitation outcome is seen by some as a reflection of biological as well as social factors (Hogarty, 1985; Flor-Henry, 1990). Problems in outcome have been ascribed to a combination of left-hemisphere vulnerability and more developmental disabilities in males in general, and to reduced left-hemispheric blood flow specifically in schizophrenia (Weinberger et al., 1986). Hogarty suggests that challenges to left-hemisphere integrity, reflected in task stress and implied or real criticism of performance, may precipitate more psychotic episodes and symptom exacerbations in schizophrenic men than in women. Women appear to be less hemispherically specialized and perhaps more bilateral and adaptable (Goy & McEwan, 1980). These issues suggest that the phenomenon of "high expressed emotion" (Anderson et al., 1986), in which perceived criticism and/or intrusiveness precipitate symptoms, is not limited to family transactions. They should generate questions about currently accepted rehabilitation techniques and therapist-patient interactions, as well as underscoring the need for feasible goals and treatment strategies that reflect greater understanding of the biopsychosocial issues in schizophrenia.

These issues provide an extemely important context for the work of rehabilitation specialists, with respect to the possible etiologies of particularly tenacious symptoms and behaviors, and should focus and intensify treatment and research efforts. The presence of structural and neurochemical brain abnormalities should not be used to preclude potentials for functional change, but rather to promote well-conceived interventions and studies that acknowledge the biological, psychological and social nature of behavior and the need for interactive, rather than unidimensional, approaches.

The Bio-Psycho-Social Model

The development of brain-behavioral paradigms for schizophrenia has piqued the interest of those who believe that function and role performance are mediated by the interaction of biological, psychological, social, and environmental factors. The Diathesis-Stress Interaction Model (DSI) for schizophrenia brings together what are often disparate perspectives of human behavior.

DSI views schizophrenic patients' difficulties in the context of their neurobiological and affective capacities, the demands of a given role and task, and the expectations and dynamics of the social-environmental press (Fine, in press). Symptoms arise when an individual with preexisting areas of vulnerability (i.e., a brain disorder) is confronted with life stressors when the valence between stressor and problem-solving capacity is unevenly matched (Zubin & Spring, 1977). Low thresholds for disorganization in such individuals further contribute to vulnerability, while internal and environmental stressors increase arousal and produce competing responses. Stressors impinging on the patient's social network appear to be the most powerful and disruptive. Withdrawal, inattention, poor judgment, anger, and florid symptoms often erupt in response to these processes.

Gazzaniga's view (1988) of schizophrenia as "a disease that finds the brain's interpreter (left hemisphere) going wild in its attempts to bring order out of what is most likely endogenous, or inner-generated, brain chaos" (p. 74) captures the essence of the situation. The task of diminishing that chaos is a daunting but crucial one. DSI provides a useful frame of reference for understanding the complex nature of performance problems: the adequacy of fit between the task and interpersonal demands of the environment and the underlying cognitive, affective, and social capacities of the individual have an effect on response, compliance, and outcome.

Perhaps DSI's greatest value lies in the attention it gives to cognitive capacity and control, the role cognition plays in mediating and managing daily living, and the role it should assume in the development of a more effective range of interactive treatment initiatives.

Cognitive Rehabilitation

Brain-behavioral models of schizophrenia make a compelling case for treatment strategies that address "brain chaos" by first focusing on inadequate capacities for information processing (i.e., attention, visual processing, organization, problem solving, judgment, cognitive flexibility) and for self monitoring; only after such consideration should treatment embark upon more complex and demanding social-interpersonal transactions and specific areas of role performance such as work. If brain impairment is a contributing factor in the persistent deficit behaviors of schizophrenia, cognitive rehabilitation techniques traditionally used to generate more efficient function in the traumatically brain-injured should be put to the test with those patients in whom negative symptoms predominate (Carpenter et al., 1985; Magaro et al., 1986; Spaulding et al., 1986, 1989). Although "one cannot assume equivalency of brain injuries acquired by trauma with the seemingly longer term anomalies of schizophrenia, theories of neuroplasticity, work with the learning-disabled, and reports of functional gains in stroke patients long after the traditional window of opportunity for recovery has closed, provide food for thought" (Fine, in press).

Cognitive rehabilitation focuses on the infrastructure of thought and action. It systematically stimulates and organizes capacities to handle information by improving mental strategies and developing behavioral repertoires with which to learn, perceive, and interact appropriately with the environment (Abreu & Toglia, 1987). It presumes that brain damage does not necessarily eliminate the complete capacity to perform a task. Efficiency may be diminished, but the brain provides a variety of means for function to occur. Luria's (1963, 1973, 1980) approach to the reorganization of functional systems in the brain-injuried is based upon a belief in the adaptive potential of the cortical system in interaction with the environment over time. Motivation, meaningful activity, and conscious compensation are critical contributors to such adaptation (Armstrong, 1989). Luria's retraining methods involved systematic repetitive exercises of increasing complexity that served to stimulate more adequate performance of impaired skills. This approach has influenced several generations of cognitive specialists, although it is not the only model in use. A variety of perspectives on cognitive rehabilitation of the brain-injured can be found in Bach-y-Rita (1990), Ben-Yishay and Diller (1983), Dougherty and Randomski (1987), Meier et al. (1987), Prigatono (1985), Sohlberg and Mateer (1989), Toglia (1989a, 1989b, 1990, 1991), and Trexler (1987).

APPLICATIONS TO MENTAL ILLNESS

Carpenter et al. (1985) have acknowledged the potential relevance of cognitive rehabilitation for patients with primary residual deficits, suggesting the use of formalized problem-solving strategies to develop graded solutions to complex tasks, feedback that helps identify consequence of incorrect solutions, exercises that develop cognitive flexibility, and programs that provide guidance for regulating behaviors that ordinarily rely on frontal lobe integrity.

Spaulding and associates (1986, 1989) present an appealing framework for cognitive interventions at the "molecular level" that incorporates concerns for vulnerability, stress, information-processing overload, hyperarousal, and social-interpresonal deficits. They focus rehabilitation on reducing arousal from levels that produce acute disorganization; raising the threshold for disorganization; and providing environmental conditions and learning experiences that favor organization. Brenner (1987, 1988) underscores the relationships among molecular and molar functional levels (attentional/perceptual, cognitive, micro-social and macro-social) and has developed integrated training techniques that address all of these areas. Although the general fund of descriptive and research data about such applications to schizophrenia is limited, greater interest is being reported at professional conferences and in the literature (Brown et al., 1991; Delahunty et al., 1991; Fine & Weiden, 1985; Fine, 1990; Fine & Toglia, 1990, 1991; Frost et al., 1991; Magaro, 1986; Olbrich & Mussgay, 1990).

Task-Oriented Learning Therapy

The particular application of cognitive rehabilitation described here incorporates the work of occupational therapists in the Departments of Rehabilitation Medicine and Psychiatry at New York Hospital–Cornell University Medical Center, NYH-CUMC (Fine, in press; Fine & Schwimmer, 1986; Greenberg et al., 1986; Toglia, 1991, 1992; Toglia & Golisz, 1990). An integrated treatment package, called Task Oriented Learning Therapy (TOLT), addresses information processing, self-monitoring capacities, and social-interpersonal skills in one-to-one and group treatment formats based upon individual readiness for changing stimuli. A range of selected graded treatment activities, staged in a variety of progressively demanding environments, are used to strengthen basic cognitive skills, processing streategies, metacognitive capacities, and social competencies. Treatment modalities include computer and tabletop games and exercises, functional tasks performed in the clinic and the community, and a psychoeducational group program called the Life Skills Curriculum.

The overall goal of this treatment program is to enhance the efficiency and flexibility of responses to the demands of clinical and natural environments. The TOLT package, usually offered in combination with medication, is planned on the basis of assessments of functional deficits, strengths, potentials, motivation, and life context.* It is designed to be responsive to biological vulnerabilities, high arousal potentials, cognitive deficits, and low thresholds for disorganization, as well as to the patient's personal goals and priorities for daily living. The challenge of transferring skills learned within the treatment setting to the demands of everyday living is of particular import and is addressed by the multicontext approach (Toglia 1991).

*Although this chapter does not elaborate on the functional assessment process, it is viewed as an essential component of treatment planning and ongoing monitoring of treatment responses. The author believes that traditional deficit-centered neuropsychological methods alone are inadequate for guiding treatment and estimating potential for change—particularly for schizophrenic patients whose deficits often obscure other attributes. Rehabilitation specialists also need to know how patients organize new information, how quickly they learn and how long they retain it, how they make decisions in the presence of environmental demands, and how accurately they evaluate their own performance. The reader is therefore referred to Toglia's (1989a) work on a dynamic investigative approach to assessment and to the AOTA Self Study Series: Assessing Function (Royeen, 1989) for a fuller exploration of functional performance and a multidimensional person-task-environment approach to the assessment process.

THE MULTICONTEXT APPROACH

Problems in the generalization of acquired skills to everyday life have undermined the benefits of many promising treatment methods for both mentally ill and brain-injured individuals. In attacking this problem, Toglia (1991, 1992) has applied contemporary cognitive psychology concepts of learning to the problem of skills transfer and generalization in the brain-injured through the use of multicontext strategies. Following assessment methods that identify deficits, strengths, and factors that maximize performance, she formulates treatment plans that focus on one or two processing and metacognitive deficiencies. For example, for a patient whose attentional deficits are reflected in tendencies to overfocus on details, thereby limiting information with which to size up situations accurately, the processing streategy of choice may be searching for information in a planned, systematic manner. This approach, along with self-monitoring training to enhance awareness of problems in performance, will be the constant factors in the treatment process. However, the environment, motor requirements, and physical and interpersonal characteristics of the treatment task will be gradually altered. A series of tasks (including tabletop exercises and games, computer activities, and simulated and real activities of daily living that reflect individual interests) will be graded to decrease physical and conceptual similarities with the initial treatment task. A detailed task analysis is used to select a sequence of activities that gradually diminishes in similarity of surface characteristics while requiring the constant application of the targeted processing and self-monitoring strategies. This method is designed to facilitate the transfer of learning by focusing attention on the core, rather than surface, attributes of tasks and by demonstrating a range of circumstances in which the patient can use a given strategy.

These concepts and methods are also being applied to ambulatory schizophrenic patients involved in TOLT. In this setting, computer-generated activities, games, functional tasks, community applications, and specially designed social skills development groups are integrated components of the treatment process. The group represents yet another context in which process strategies and self-monitoring skills can be practiced. As we in mental health practice recognize the problems inherent in the heavy use of group treatments for many schizophrenic patients and look to more individualized cognitive strategies to first strengthen basic foundation skills, brain-injury specialists are seeking group treatments that consolidate gains made in individualized cognitive rehabilitation (Toglia & Golisz, 1990). Both patient populations pose difficult problems in the activation and processing of necessary cognitive and social-interpersonal capacities, and both require progressive and continuing reinforcement in multiple environments. The special attributes of the cognitive rehabilitation and social skills development components of TOLT are discussed below.

COMPUTER-BASED SKILLS ACQUISITION

The CBSA is one of several treatment modalities used in Task Oriented Learning Therapy to strengthen processing and self-monitoring capacities and to prepare patients for more cognitively and interpersonally demanding group interventions and activites of daily living in the community. Software programs involving exercises, games, and situational simulations graded to meet individual needs are used several times a week for periods dictated by patient response patterns. While these goals are also stimulated with tabletop formats and actual tasks of daily living, the popularity and unique attributes of the computer and the carefully selected software appear to enhance the treatment process. The highly interactive but modifiable nature of the computer gives patients external support needed to develop independent work habits. It provides feedback through both visual and auditory cues and can be programmed to be responsive to changing capacities. Selected software permits graded levels of difficulty in a given task based upon the complexity of the stimulus, the speed required for a response, and the availability of a variety of cues and prompts. Patients, therefore, have more control over what and how much goes on in the treatment session. Goals of personal control and self-management are also fostered by programs that provide ongoing feedback to predict and evaluate one's own performance.

Although the therapist plays a very important role in designing and directing treatment, inducting the patient into the world of high tech, introducing new tasks that apply the skill of concern in varying contexts, and adding ongoing reinforcement and support, the interpersonal demands of this intervention are far more controllable than other one-to-one and group endeavors. For many schizophrenic patients, this less-stressful task condition makes possible learning of new or different cognitive skills and mental strategies.

During the process of developing a library of appropriate software for the NYH-CUMC rehabilitation program, patients participated in the screening and selection of games, exercises, and simulations from a pool of software commonly used in special education and rehabilitation and also by the general public. They were asked to rate each on a range of task parameters. Increased motivation and self-esteem were observed among those actively contributing to the development of this and other treatment strategies. If curiosity and laughter are any measure of goodness of fit, the patient evaluators have important needs met as they review the sublime and the ridiculous in commercial software.

THE LIFE SKILLS CURRICULUM

The Life Skills Curriculum (LSC) is introduced as improvement in foundation skills appear to be maximized. In most instances, two session of cognitive rehabilitation are supplemented with one LSC session each week. The LSC uses social learning principles and graded, goal-directed tasks to cultivate problem-solving and communication skills in a small group setting (Greenberg et al., 1985; Fine & Schimmer, 1986), where participants practice the same process and self-monitoring strategies addressed in one-to-one sessions. In a classroom milieu, multimodal educational techniques—lectures, group discussion, role playing, homework assignments, notebooks, paper-and-pencil exercises, and audiovisual materials—engage visual, auditory, and motor capacities to facilitate skill acquisition. Instructional components are selected and graded to match attention, memory, and learning styles as closely as possible within a group context. As in other social-learning applications, frequent practice, repetition, reinforcement, modeling, and feedback are critical tools for fostering desired behaviors.

Although the manifest content of a class or series of classes may be goal setting, stress and time management, leisure-time planning, or social skills development, enhanced problem-solving and communication and targeted processing and self-monitoring skills are core objectives for all sessions. Participants are repeatedly reminded of the relationships between their personal goals and the content and process of the sessions. In fact, they participate in decision making at several levels about what, when, and how personal and group goals are implemented. Pre- and postcourse self-assessments support the central assumption that participants are capable of identifying their own learning needs and monitoring changes in their own behavior. The clinician's role is hardly extinguished, however, since task parameters that facilitate generalization of learning require expertise in task analysis, design, and application. The sometimes conflicting goals of expanding patients' self-management capacities and operationalizing clinician skill place special demands on the therapist's insight, sensitivity, and therapeutic use of self.

How do these things get put together? The components of Task Oriented Learning Therapy and the multicontext model for cognitive rehabilitation for schizophrenia are best conveyed through a clinical vignette.

A CASE IN POINT: THE STORY OF HELEN

Helen is a 42-year-old single high-school graduate diagnosed with chronic schizophrenia with paranoid and depressive features. The diathesis-stress model could well have been inspired by Helen. Her vulnerabilities are evident in a family history of mental illness, a personal history of physical illnesses including malaria, childhood seizures, early onset of emotional problems, and a physical demeanor that speaks of years of stigma and despair. Stress is no stranger to her. Family life has been marked with conflict, criticism, and erratic communication. Helen has so skillfully internalized these conflicts that she replays the endless stressors of the past as if they were of the moment, while often viewing present situations as if they were literally scenes from the past. Her internal conflict, along with the real daily challenges of life in an urban center, elicits high levels of arousal and disorganization that sometimes yield bizarre behaviors. Nonetheless, she is articulate, altruistic, and tenacious in her desire to function more effectively. Her many intact intellectual capacities and her ability to establish and maintain alliances with several clinicians over the years have contributed to her achievements during her best periods of function and to her survival during the worst of times.

Helen has experienced many brief hospitalizations, outpatient treatment with a variety of practitioners and programs, a compromised work history and social network, and inadequate living conditions. Her florid symptoms are currently managed by a psychiatrist through considerable doses of medication. Her functional deficits and efforts at independent living are the focus of work with an occupational therapist in a small individualized rehabilitation program in a major medical center.

Helen's involvement with TOLT, and her many contributions to the development of this strategy, emerged from growing evidence that state-of-the-art medication, empathic talk, participation in a work program and in a social skills training group at a highly lauded psychosocial club program were *not* making a sufficient difference. She experienced rejection and isolation amid the demands of large groups of disturbed patients, and she felt flooded by contact with a changing cast of staff members. This in turn stimulated Helen's suspicious nature. In other than therapeutic situations, good performance and motivation appeared task-specific and did not protect her from the unpredictable demands of life outside the treatment center. While Helen lives alone, travels independently, handles her own limited finances, and has a good fund of knowledge, she is slow, easily overwhelmed, and frequently has difficulty in applying her knowledge and other strengths to many aspects of daily living.

Observation and patient reports centered on her extreme slowness in completing routine tasks of daily living, anxiety about trying new things, and a marked tendency to misread social cues. Formal assessment, which included neuropsychological testing and dynamic interactional methods (Toglia 1992) confirmed the presence of specific attentional and problem-solving deficits that contributed to her dysfunction. Prominent deficits were a tendency to overfocus on parts of a given task, impaired ability to consider two or more sources of information at once, and related difficulties in distinguishing critical facts from personal assumptions during problem-solving tasks. She was responsive to cuing and able to apply feedback to other situations within several assessment sessions, suggesting higher potentials for performance. Although Helen often found fault in the environment for the problems she encountered and was usually guarded in acknowledging the extent of her personal difficulties, she demonstrated basic awareness of many of her problems in thinking and doing during the assessment phase. She was able to correct her own errors with some frequency, but felt helpless in dealing with them as they occurred on a daily basis. Motivation to change and to gain more control over thought processes and behavior was noted, as was her particular interest in the educational format of the treatment program—all factors favoring learning and behavioral change.

Treatment goals, determined in collaboration with Helen, initially focused on developing abilities to attend to all relevant aspects of a task at a reasonable pace without getting stuck on single elements or on her inner thoughts. Self-monitoring training was directed at focusing her attention on predicting how long a task would take, increasing her abilities to identify when she was running into difficulty before she became irreversibly "stuck," and evaluating herself at the conclusion of tasks. These particular strategies were selected because they were basic to her concerns about her performance in self-care and home management, as well as her tendencies to ruminate over perceived injustices and to interpret social interactions from an extremely limited and biased array of information.

A series of tasks related to her interests and values were identified, analyzed, and prepared so that task characteristics (surface appearance, movement requirements, environment, and complexity) could be graded and changed along a continuum of near-to-intermediate-to-far skills transfer. The contemporary appeal of the computer, her long-time love of card games, and her interest in cooking provided sufficiently meaningful activities to construct a rich repertoire of graded treatment tasks that took her from the screen of the computer, to the card table, to cookbooks, to the supermarket and the kitchen, and to many places in between. The furthest and most meaningful transfer of skills occurred in her volunteer work placement, her home, and other aspects of community life. While the treatment tasks and characteristics changed, the targeted processing and self-monitoring strategies remained constant. Personalized cue cards, self-evaluation questionnaires, and progress graphs strengthened her abilities to predict and measure her own performance, both within and outside of sessions. After improvement in her abilities to focus and control attention to problem solving in increasingly complex and different tasks, she joined a group of five other patients with comparable cognitive difficulties in the Life Skills Curriculum. Group sessions, focused on problem-solving and communication skills, also provided more challenging opportunities to fortify the pace and efficiency of her mental strategies and metacognitive skills within a social-interpersonal milieu. Multimodal tasks were used here as well, but within a classroom format. Treatment objectives were put into action through group activities, games, video exercises, guided role playing, and focused discussions, reinforced with homework assignments. Even planning for the group's refreshments provided opportunities to incorporate desired skills while collaborating with others. Because individual goals are shared within the group, solicited and unsolicited feedback from peers serves as another perspective or source of reinforcement. Helen's ability to use these strategies with greater efficiency in functional tasks involving things rather than people was obvious. Nonetheless, in encounters within the group and with salespeople in her neighborhood, she was more frequently able to internalize the goal of considering all the relevant facts before "getting stuck" or "jumping to upsetting conclusions." Individual and group modalities were used concurrently for several months until

Helen's comfort and performance levels stabilized and the supervisors at her volunteer worksite asked her to increase her hours with them. The patient and her therapists perceived this to be the best of all outcome measures. Individual and group sessions, referred to as "continuing education," were used twice monthly to identify problems in daily living and to reinforce skills.

* * *

Reports in the literature (Delahunty et al., 1991) and the author's experience demonstrate that what constitutes an adequate "dose" of this kind of treatment varies greatly among individuals. Helen's good response to strategies that facilitated processing and self-monitoring capacities around predictable activities of daily living was reasonably rapid. Application to more unpredictable life events, however, posed another level of skill transfer that required additional, ongoing interventions. For this patient, engagement and progress were decidedly positive, although highly dependent upon the degree to which she was exposed to family stressors and able to ignore them by internalizing her otherwise external locus of control. Other patients with deficit symptoms who are less accessible and less motivated require longer trials because of the complexity of their deficits, their difficulties in establishing or maintaining a reasonable therapeutic alliance, and their need for small, manageable skill increments and repeated opportunities for practice and reinforcement in multiple contexts.

* * *

This chapter's efforts to put skills acquisition into proper perspective is based upon a belief in the interactive nature of social competency and role competency. Biological, psychological, and socioenvironmental factors all contribute to the functional successes and failures of our patients. However, special emphasis must be placed on the importance of the cognitive infrastructure and the need to look beneath manifest behaviors if one is to understand and promote functional change. The complex problems that beseige those with chronic mental illness defy unidimensional approaches. Graded skills acquisition, directed at the optimal match between levels of function and levels of arousal (Kaplan, 1988), when presented at the patient's pace and reflective of the person's interests and values, is most likely to yield sustained engagement and adaptive responses. Multicontext methods, like the Task Oriented Learning Therapy package (along with appropriate doses of medication), appear to hold great promise. Research initiatives to evaluate the efficacy of this approach are underway. The results will be the most compelling proof of the value of these efforts for this challenging group of patients and for the cognitive rehabilitation movement in mental health.

Cognitive Rehabilitation and the Mental Health System

The values, expertise, and commitments of individual treatment programs flourish or falter within the larger context of local, state, and national systems of health care and human services. Even as researchers and clinicians move closer to a fuller understanding of the interactive nature of the schizophrenic process and the interventions that foster the integration of biopsychosocial phenomena, most health care systems are limiting access to services through regulation, reimbursement restrictions, managed care, and unenlightened neglect. The well-documented failings of deinstitutionalization in the 1960s and current practices intended to contain costs are powerful examples of the ways "the system" separates those in need from relevant services. Mechanic (1991) suggests that these failings occur because of "dispersion of responsibility and authority, the lack of professional incentives, perverse financial inducements, the bureaucratization of care, the influence of entrenched groups, legal obstacles, and a lack of interest among influential public officials" (p. 797).

Rehabilitation specialists and advocates, not unlike the chronic patients they champion, have often found rehabilitation derailed or ignored by the system—viewed as "the fourth leg of medical practice" (Hinsie & Campbell, 1970), something that possibly occurs after diagnosis, treatment, and prevention. Although important gains have been made in reconciling such distortions and in fostering a more collaborative partnership between medical and rehabilitation models, many rehabilitation practitioners continue to experience themselves (and their domain of interest) as outsiders. Those who have brought their programs out of the basements (real and symbolic) of state hospitals, university services, and community settings have often been confronted by disorganized or uninterested systems. The significant funding and visibility of such programs as Fountain House in New York and the skills training modules disseminated by Liberman and Anthony and colleagues attest to the fact that in some circumstances the system *can* be engaged.

Some innovative programs for the chronically mentally ill have emerged in spite of the absence of substantive support from the larger system. Such "heroics" (perceived as such by researchers who function under the auspices of significant funding) are often productive and satisfying, but frequently fade or fail to fulfill their potential when longer-term support does not materialize. This has been the plight of some seemingly sound but untested cognitive interventions developed by committed clinicians who needed, but did not get, mentoring, access to research knowhow, "permission" to use some of their time for new and different activities, or the collegiality of other professionals with similar commitments. These resources constitute a system too, albeit not the one we have learned to blame for all the failures in health care.

The NYH-CUMC cognitive rehabilitation strategy has emerged from a grassroots system. This project, evolving through various formats over the past seven years, has been fueled principally by personal commitment and by the diverse human and material resources of a teaching hospital where such activity is valued. In addition, startup grant support was received from the American Occupational Therapy Foundation for the earlier development of the Life Skills Curriculum component. Psychiatrist colleagues have also provided support and have joined us in developing research protocols designed to test the efficacy of this treatment package. The patients and their families also represent a contributing component of this system. They are not simply subjects of technology development but active, knowledgeable collaborators, judging the fit between our evolving interventions and their potentials to learn and change. In fact, funding for computer equipment came from the family of one of the patients.

However, even in the relatively well-endowed academic sector many clinical, administrative, political, and economic factors discourage the focused thoughts and persistent behaviors needed to develop, operationalize, evaluate, and refine new treatment streategies. Among them are the unpredictable changes within a facility that alter access to patients and staff, equally unpredictable changes within individual patients that make them less available, and very predictable interprofessional tensions that arise from differences in perspective and priorities. For this project, the task of sorting out the many disparate schools of thought about cognition and of selecting language that can be meaningfully shared has been particularly challenging. As frustrating and time-consuming as these tasks are, they have been offset by the stimulation inherent in such problem-solving endeavors.

What can be expected from the mental health system once the NYH-CUMC program is refined and packaged and has generated preliminary data on effectiveness? It is difficult to say. Certainly all professional activities are shadowed by the realities of serious financial problems. Much depends on the kind of research and service that today's market will buy and on how skillfully we present our products. Will the highly individualized nature of multicontext treatment and other cognitive rehabilitation strategies "fit" traditional large-scale research methods? Do we design protocols that are guided by standard psychometric procedures that are acceptable to funding sources even if they may not reflect the unique nature of our treatment (Carpenter, 1991)? What kinds of treatment will we be able to provide for seriously impaired individuals in 40 annual reimbursable outpatient visits? Do we design treatment to meet the needs of the patient or the resources of the system? Is cognitive technology too esoteric and time-intensive to appeal to state mental health office personnel and Medicaid surveyors? These are but a few of the political-ethical-career conundrums that come with the territory and will continue to influence work on programs like Task Oriented Learning Therapy.

THE NEW YORK STATE PLAN: WHERE THERE'S LIFE THERE'S HOPE

Despite many discouraging factors, there are some conceptual and procedural changes in the New York State Office of Mental Health (OMH) regulations that may provide interesting opportunities for rehabilitation professionals, consumers, and their advocates. Similar changes may emerge in other states as well. New program initiatives, tied to state-controlled reimbursement incentives and deterrents, emphasize timely, intensive, functionally oriented aftercare services for the chronically mentally ill. OMH regulations place special emphasis on rehabilitation strategies that promote a consumer-empowering philosophy, that value patients' views of their own needs, and that cultivate motivation, role performance, and overall community adaptation (New York State OMH, 1990). These are words that warm the heart of the most jaded practitioners, even in the face of a budgetary crisis that has already undermined many of the values and guidelines. But these words also need to be examined with care. While they reflect very important psychosocial rehabilitation concepts and they acknowledge the need for transfer of learning from clinic to community, the models from which these initiatives have emerged (Farkas & Anthony, 1988) consider "skill acquisition" only at the levels of social skills and social roles—*not* from cognitive or information-processing perspectives. The NYH-CUMC Life Skills Curriculum fits the OMH prescription, but cognitive rehabilitation strategies are not specifically mentioned by OMH and therefore may well fall between the regulatory and reimbursement cracks.

To avoid such a possibility, proposals have been submitted for optional services that would qualify for state reimbursement. Proposals such as these define and describe cognitive approaches and the rationale for their availability and funding. Such efforts create important opportunities to educate health planners about the nature of human performance and the functional deficits linked with schizophrenia, and about why medication, behavioral treatments, and support systems may not be adequate for many patients. Increased visibility of cognitive strategies in governmental and advocacy sectors must occur concurrently with technology development and assessment if bureaucratic barriers are to be breached and professional incentives cultivated. Resilient as that plan of action may seem, it does represent yet another task added to the already overloaded agenda of those who develop programs and who want to see their ideas and efforts disseminated and validated.

Conclusion

The neuroscientific trends of the past two decades, as well as growing interdisciplinary interest in the interaction among central nervous system, environment, and illness, hold great promise for stimulating more effective treatment and rehabilitation for schizophrenia. We have an expanding scientific base and emerging opportunities for increasing our understanding of patients' failures to function and our failures to rehabilitate.

Gazzaniga (1988) aptly captures the challenge of schizophrenia when he calls it a powerful model of "the fate of the human mind when exposed to long-term distortions of reality" (p. 89). He suggests that our task is to develop a framework that ties together brain abnormalities, the personal psychological reality of the mind, and its capacities to fulfill a person's potential in a given environment. This idea should guide our efforts to develop responsive rehabilitation technology. Our collective interest in cognition represents a crucial link, bridging bio-psycho-social sectors of performance and adaptation. Individuals committed to this task must seize the opportunity for systematic thought and action in both clinical and research endeavors.

However, the strength of these patient-centered and academic commitments must not diminish our responsibilities to the larger system. Mental health specialists know all too well that issues of access, quality, and outcome are of great importance. They represent major challenges to the durability of our efforts. We must not ignore the history of rehabilitation and society's shifting social, political, and economic trends. We must meet the ebb and flow of interest in rehabilitation and the chronically mentally ill with stronger and more effective partnerships among colleagues, government, advocacy groups, patients, and the communities in which they live. Only then will we be abel to put the needs of our patients and the promise of cognitive rehabilitation into proper perspective.

References

Abreu, B., & Toglia, J. P. (1987). Cognitive rehabilitation: A model for occupational therapy. *American Journal of Occupational Therapy,* 41, 439–448.

Anderson, C. M., Reiss, D. J., & Hogarty, G. E. (1986). *Schizophrenia and the family.* New York: Guilford Press.

Andreason, N. (1982a). Negative symptoms in schizophrenia: Definition and reliability. *Archives of General Psychiatry,* 39, 784–788.

Andreason, N. (1982b). Negative vs. positive schizophrenia: Definition and validation. *Archives of General Psychiatry,* 39, 789–94.

Andreason, N. (1983). *The scale for the assessment of negative symptoms (SANS).* Iowa City: University of Iowa Press.

Andreason, N. (1985). Positive vs. negative schizophrenia: A critical evaluation. *Schizophrenia Bulletin,* 11(3), 380–389.

Anthony, W. A., & Liberman, R. P. (1986). The practice of psychiatric rehabilitation: Historical, conceptual and research base. *Schizophrenia Bulletin,* 12(4), 542–559.

Armstrong, C. (1989). Luria's theory of brain function recovery with applications to the use of computers in cognitive retraining. *Cognitive Rehabilitation* Jan./Feb. 10–15.

Bach-y-Rita, P. (1980). Brain plasticity as a basis for therapeutic procedures. In P. Bach-y-Rita, (Ed.), *Recovery of function: Theoretical considerations for brain injury rehabilitation.* Bern: Hans Huber.

Ben-Yishay, Y., & Diller, L. (1983). Cognitive remediation. In M. Rosenthal (Ed.), *Rehabilitation of the head injured adult.* Philadelphia: F. A. Davis Co.

Ben-Yishay, Y., Piasetsky, E. B., & Ratlok, K. S. (1987). A systematic method for ameliorating disorders in basic attention. In M. J. Meier, A. L. Benton, & L. Diller (Eds.), *Neuropsychological rehabilitation.* London: Churchill Livingstone.

Brenner, H. D. (1987). On the importance of cognitive disorders in treatment and rehabilitation. In J. S. Strauss, W. Boker, & H. D. Brenner (Eds.), *Psychosocial treatment of schizophrenia.* Bern: Hans Huber.

Brenner, H. D., Kraemer, S., Hermanutz, M., & Hodel, B. (1988). Cognitive treatment in schizophrenia. In E. Straube & H. Halweg (Eds.), *Schizophrenia: Models and interventions.* Heidelberg: Springer.

Brown, C., Hays, C., Short, J., & Harwood K. (1991, June). Applying neuroscience to mental health practice. Paper presented at the American Occupational Therapy Association Annual Meeting, Cincinnati.

Carpenter, W. T. (1991). Editorial: Psychopathology and common sense. *Biological Psychiatry,* 29, 735–737.

Carpenter, W. T., Heinrichs, D. W., & Alphs, S. D. (1985). Treatment of negative symptoms. *Schizophrenia Bulletin,* 11(3), 440–452.

Carpenter, W. T., Strauss, J. S., & Bartko, J. J. (1973). Flexible system for the diagnosis of schizophrenia: Report from the WHO International Pilot Study of Schizophrenia. *Science,* 182, 1275–1277.

Christianson, C. (1991). Occupational therapy: Intervention for life performance. In C. Christianson & C. Baum (Eds.), *Occupational therapy: Overcoming human performance deficits.* Thorofare, N.J.: Slack Inc.

Delahunty, A., Morice, R., Frost, B., & Lambert, F. (1991). Neurocognitive rehabilitation in schizophrenia eight years post–head injury: A case study. *Cognitive Rehabilitation,* 9(5), 24–28.

Dougherty, P. M., & Randomski, M. V. (1987). *Cognitive rehabilitation workbook.* Rockville, Md.: Aspen Publishers.

Fine, S. B. (1980). Psychiatric treatment and rehabilitation: What's in a name? *Psychiatric Hospital,* 12, 8–13.

Fine, S. B. (1990, Feb. 7). Reframing rehabilitation: The influence of differential therapeutics, neuroscience and time. Presentation at Connecticut Mental Health Center, New Haven.

Fine, S. B. (1990, May 17). Task oriented learning for deficit symptoms: Putting skill acquisition into proper perspective. Proc. Symposium: Treatment of negative symptoms of schizophrenia. American Psychiatric Association 143d Annual Meeting, New York City.

Fine, S. B. (in press). Neurobehavioral perspectives on schizophrenia. In J. Van Duesen (Ed.), *Rehabilitation of adults with perceptual-motor dysfunction.* Orlando, Fla.: W. B. Saunders Co.

Fine, S. B., & Schwimmer, P. (1986). The effects of occupational therapy on independent living skills. *Mental Health Special Interest Newsletter* (American Occupational Therapy Association), 9, 1–3.

Fine, S. B., & Toglia, J. P. (1990, November 3). Applying cognitive rehabilitation to mental health practice: Assessment and treatment streategies for schizophrenia. Paper presented at conference, New York Hospital–Cornell University Mendical Center, New York City.

Fine, S. B., & Toglia, J. P. (1991, March). Applying cognitive rehabilitation to mental health practice: Assessment and treatment streategies for schizophrenia. Paper presented at conference, Institute of The Pennsylvania Hospital, Philadelphia.

Fine, S. B., & Toglia, J. P. (1991, June). Applying cognitive rehabilitation to mental health practice: Assessment and treatment streategies for schizophrenia. Paper presented at workshop, American Occupational Therapy Association Annual Meeting, Cincinnati.

Fine, S. B., & Weiden, P. (1985). Adapting the rehabilitation model: Phase-specific approaches to the negative symptoms of schizophrenia. Paper presented at Institute of Hospital & Community Psychiatry, Boston.

Flor-Henry, P. (1990). Influence of gender in schizophrenia as related to other psychopathological syndromes. *Schizophrenia Bulletin,* 16(2), 211–227.

Frost, B., Morice, R. D., Delahunty, A., Gulliver, S., Ryan, M., Framptom, G., Connolly, S., & Hunter, M. (1991). Neurocognitive and psychosocial rehabilitation of chronic schizophrenia: A clinical study. In W. Levick, B. Frost, M. Watson, & P. Pfister (Eds.), *Brain impairment: Advances in applied research.* Newcastle: University of Newcastle.

Gazzaniga, M. S. (1988). *Mind matters: How mind and brain interact to create our conscious lives.* Boston: Houghton Mifflin.

Gibson, J. J. (1986). *The ecological approach to visual perception.* Hillsdale, N.Y.: Lawrence Erlbaum Associates.

Goy, R. W., & McEwen, B. S. (1980). *Sexual differentiation of the brain.* Cambridge: MIT Press.

Greenberg, L., Fine, S. B., Cohen, C., Larson, K., Michaelson-Baily, A., Rubinton, P., & Glick, I. (1986). An interdisciplinary psychoeducational program for schizophrenic patients and their families in an acute care setting. *Hospital & Community Psychiatry* 39(3), 277–282.

Gritzer, G., & Arluke, A. (1985). *The Making of rehabilitation: A political economy of medical specialization, 1890–1980.* Berkeley: University of California Press.

Hinsie, L. E., & Campbell, R. J. (1970). *Psychiatric dictionary.* 4th ed. London: Oxford University Press.

Hogarty, G. E. (1985, October). Treatment resistance of schizophrenic patients to social and vocational rehabilitation: The nature of the problem and model of treatment. Paper presented at International Symposium on Schizophrenia, Munich.

Holtzman, P. S. (1985). Eye movement dysfunctions and psychosis. *International Review of Neurobiology,* 27, 179–205.

Kaplan, K. (1988). *Directive group therapy.* Thorofare, N.J.: Slack, Inc.

Koh, S. D. (1978). Remembering verbal materials by schizophrenic young adults. In

S. Schwartz (Ed.), *Language and cognition in schizophrenia.* Hillsdale, N.J.: Erlbaum.

Leigh, R. J., & Zee, D. S. (1983). *The neurology of eye movements.* Philadelphia: FA Davis Co.

Liberman, R. P. (Ed.) (1988). *Psychiatric rehabilitation of chronic mental patients.* Washington, D.C.: American Psychiatric Press.

Luria, A. R. (1973). The frontal lobes and the regulation of behavior. In K. Pribram & A. R. Luria (Eds.), *The psychophysiology of the frontal lobes.* New York: Academic Press.

Luria, A. R. (1980). *Higher cortical functions in man.* New York: Basic Books.

Luria, A. R. (1963). *Restoration of function after brain injury.* New York: Macmillan Co.

Magaro, P. A., Johnson, M. H., & Boring, R. (1986). Information processing approaches to the treatment of schizophrenia. In R. Ingram (Ed.), *Information processing approaches to clinical psychology.* New York: Academic Press.

Mayer, M. A. (1988). Analysis of information processing and cognitive disability theory. *American Journal of Occupational Therapy,* 42(3), 176–183.

McGhie, A., Chapman, J., & Lawson, J. S. (1965). The effect of distraction on schizophrenic performance: 2. Psychomotor ability. *British Journal of Psychiatry,* 111, 391–40.

McGrath, M. E. (1984). First person accounts: Where did I go? *Schizophrenia Bulletin,* 10, 638–640.

Mechanic, D. (1991). Strategies for integrating public mental health services. *Hospital & Community Psychiatry,* 42(8), 797–801.

Meier, M., Diller, L., & Benton, A., (Eds.) (1987). *Neuropsychological rehabilitation.* New York: Guilford Press.

Meltzer, H. (1987). Biological studies in schizophrenia. *Schizophrenia Bulletin,* 13(1), 77–111.

Meltzer, H., & Stahl, S. M. (1976). The dopamine hypothesis of schizophrenia: A review. *Schizophrenia Bulletin,* 2, 19–76.

Meyer, A. (1922). A philosophy of occupational therapy. *Archives of Occupational Therapy,* 1, 1–10.

National Institute of Mental Health. (1988). *A national plan for schizophrenia research: Report of the National Advisory Mental Health Council (*DHHS Publication no. ADM 88-1571). Rockville, Md.: NIMH.

Neuchterlein, K. H., & Dawson, M. C. (1984). Information processing and attentional functioning in the developmental course of schizophrenic disorders. *Schizophrenia Bulletin,* 10, 160–203.

Olbrich, R., & Mussgay, L. (1990). Reduction of schizophrenic deficits by cognitive training: An evaluative study. *European Archives of Psychiatry & Neurological Sciences,* 239, 366–369.

Owens, D. G., Johnstone, E. C., Crow, T. J., Frith, C. D., Jagoe, J. R., & Kreel, L.

(1985). Lateral ventricular size in schizophrenia: Relationship to the disease process and its clinical manifestations. *Psychological Medicine,* 15:27–41.

Prigatono, G. (1985). *Neuropsychological rehabilitation after brain injury.* Baltimore, Md.: Johns Hopkins University Press.

Rappaport, M., Hopkins, H. K., & Hall, K. (1972). Auditory signal detection in paranoid and nonparanoid schizophrenics. *Archives of General Psychiatry,* 27, 747–752.

Royeen, C. (Ed.) (1989). *Self-study series: Functional assessment.* Rockville, Md.: American Occupational Therapy Association.

Saccuzzo, D. P., Hirt, M., & Spencer, T. (1974). Backward masking as a measure of attention in schizophrenia. *Journal of Abnormal Psychology,* 83, 512–522.

Sohlberg, M. M., & Mateer, C. A. (1989). *Introduction to cognitive rehabilitation: Theory and practice.* New York: Guilford Press.

Spaulding, W. D., Garbin, C. P., & Crinean, W. J. (1989). The logical and psychometric prerequisites for cognitive therapy of schizophrenia. *British Journal of Psychiatry,* 155(5), 69–73.

Spaulding, W. D., Storms, L., Goodrich, V., & Sullivan, M. (1986). Experimental psychopathology in psychiatric rehabilitation. *Schizophrenia Bulletin,* 12(4), 560–577.

Toglia, J. P. (1989). Approaches to cognitive assessment of the brain injured adult: Traditional methods and dynamic investigation. *Occupational Therapy Practice* 1(1), 36–55.

Toglia, J. P. (1992). A dynamic interactional approach to cognitive rehabilitation. In N. Katz (Ed.), *Cognitive rehabilitation: Models for intervention in occupational therapy* (pp. 104–143). Boston: Andover Medical Publisher.

Toglia, J. P. (1991). Generalization of treatment: A multicontextual approach to cognitive perceptual impairment in the brain injured adult. *American Journal of Occupational Therapy,* 45(6), 505–516.

Toglia, J. P. (1989). Visual perception of objects: an approach to assessment and intervention. *American Journal of Occupational Therapy,* 44, 578–595.

Toglia, J. P., & Golisz, K. (1990). *Cognitive rehabilitation: Group games and activities.* Tucson: Therapy Skill Builders.

Trexler, L. (1982). *Cognitive rehabilitation: Conceptualization and intervention.* New York: Plenum Press.

Vezzetti, D. (1989). Capacity, content, control: A model for analyzing the cognitive demands of activity. *Occupational Therapy Practice,* 1(1), 9–17.

Weinberger, D. R., & Kleinman, J. E. (1986). Observation on the brain in schizophrenia. In R. E. Hales & A. J. Frances (Eds.), *Psychiatric update: annual review,* Vol. 5 (pp. 42–67). Washington, D.C.: American Psychiatric Association.

Wohlberg, G., & Kornetsky, C. (1973). Sustained attention in remitted schizophrenics. *Archives of General Psychiatry,* 28, 533–537.

Zubin, J., & Spring, G. (1977). Vulnerability: A new view of schizophrenia. *Journal of Abnormal Psychology,* 86, 103–126.

•7•

Clinical Rehabilitation of Schizophrenia: Development of a Theory-Based Program

M. T. Appelo, C. J. Slooff, F. M. J. Woonings,

J. W. Louwerens, M. van der Gaag,

and R. J. van den Bosch

In The Netherlands, as in most other countries, the number of patients diagnosed with schizophrenia is approximately 0.7 to 1.0 percent of the total population. In 75 percent of cases this disturbance takes a chronic form. Within 10 years after the onset of illness, around 40 percent of patients require protected living conditions, and a normal working situation is rarely possible. The suicide rate is about 9 percent (Slooff, 1988). Schizophrenic patients occupy 60 to 70 percent of beds in psychiatric hospitals. At least 30 percent of these are readmissions (Ministerie van Welzijn, Volksgezondheid en Cultuur, 1984).

These somber statistics may reflect the view of medical personnel who see their task exclusively as elimination of symptoms. Too little attention is given to the frequently chronic nature of the patients' disabilities and the fact that patients change and adapt to changed circumstances more slowly than most people. Research has shown that disability expressed in limited social role performance is prominent in 70 percent of patients (tenHorn, 1986).

The rehabilitation of schizophrenic patients is becoming a political issue, in part because the promise of social reintegration and reentry into the workforce has political consequences (Stuurgroep Toekomstscenario's Gezondheidszorg, 1990). This prominence is causing government agencies to encourage development of rehabilitation services in mental health systems, at least for the time being. However, rehabilitation is also a technological issue. If the technology cannot fulfill the promise, support for it will eventually die out. One of the problems with rehabilitation is that the theoretical basis of its technology is often absent, or is poorly developed when put into practice. The result is treatment based on inadequate diagnosis and a limited therapy repertoire, which fails to take into account individual potential and limitations. The effects of treatment are seldom adequately assessed, resulting in a lack of empirical support for its continuation or change. Thus, the importance of development, implementation, and evaluation of theoretically directed rehabilitation is great.

This chapter describes the theoretical basis of a comprehensive rehabilitation program for patients with chronic schizophrenia, developed in response to priorities set by Dutch public policy. The clinical outcome of this program is described and discussed in chapter 8 of this volume.

Theoretical Starting Points

Schizophrenia is no longer understood to be a chronic illness irrevocably associated with progressive deterioration. Longitudinal studies have shown that many schizophrenic patients' functional level reaches a plateau after five to ten years and then remains stable, sometimes resulting in fairly good outcome (Harding et al., 1987b; McGlashan, 1988). Today schizophrenia is viewed as an episodic phenomenon, with debilitating consequences, that accompanies failure of coping in vulnerable individuals (Zubin & Spring, 1977).

Wing (1978) distinguishes between fundamental primary impairments of schizophrenia, based on symptomatology and behavior, and secondary impairments. The primary impairments include basic psychological disturbances such as dysfunctions of thought and mood, disorientation, memory loss, perceptual distortions, and the immediate consequences for the patient. Secondary impairments include reactions to the presence of the primary impairments and the associated loss of role, position, and expectations for the future. These are related to fear, intractability, derangement, and denial, as well as to inadequate coping behavior. The reactions are influenced by so-called premorbid impairments, traits associated with subtle cognitive deficits, limited frustration tolerance, instability of self-esteem and object relations, and deficient practical and social skills. Wing also identifies tertiary impairments, or responses by the patient to reactions of others to the patient's disturbance. Tertiary impairments may take the form of guilt in response to disappointed family members or employers, anger, aggression, depression, or rebelliousness. Such responses bring further rejection and stigmatization.

These theoretical developments in the understanding of schizophrenia portray a complex condition, with causal factors operating across a spectrum of biological, intrapersonal, and social domains and over the course of development. Concepts such as vulnerability, cognitive deficits, stress, and coping do not figure in traditional treatment approaches. For the purposes of rehabilitation, these concepts should be systematically addressed in the course of program design and development.

A Cognitive Model for Program Development

Cognitive deficits have long been thought to be associated with schizophrenia, although it is relatively recently that such deficits have been studied scientifically. A number of measurable deficits occur in a high proportion of patients. Some are trait-like, present before onset and after remission as vulnerability factors, while others appear to come and go with psychotic episodes. Many cognitive deficits can be expected to interfere with rehabilitation, especially because of the degree to which psychiatric rehabilitation has come to rely on skill acquisition as a central mechanism for its treatment effect. Nevertheless, treatment programs for schizophrenic patients often fail to address or even recognize cognitive disturbances adequately (Bellak, Morrison & Mueser, 1989), much less consider their role in compromising skill acquisition.

Anderson's (1983) model of human cognition provides a general theoretical framework for adapting practical teaching methods to the cognitive dysfunctions of schizophrenia. According to his model, effective skills are developed through a *production system*—a programmed, step-by-step plan in which the skill comes to be performed automatically. Any skill performance reflects the functioning of a production system, and a new production system must be established if new skill acquisition is to occur. Only when a new program repeatedly takes effect does it influence behavior directly. Until then programs already present in the repertoire are used.

Production systems develop in three learning stages. Cognitive dysfunctions in schizophrenia often lead to problems in getting through these stages.

The first learning stage in Anderson's model is the *declarative stage*. Information in this stage is registered as verbal narrative, describing the behavioral steps involved in performing the skill. These steps are literally self-instructions that guide the person through unfamiliar tasks before the skill is well established. The declarative stage also includes information about the nature and importance of the skill. In this sense, it gives the skill "meaning" and thus creates motivation to acquire it.

Processing of self-instructions occurs in working memory, where it demands a large amount of cognitive capacity. In other words, while it is going on the person can simultaneously perform other processing to only a limited degree. People with schizophrenia often have deficient working memory and/or reduced cognitive capacity, so problems often occur at this stage of skill acquisition. It is therefore important for the skill trainer to make sure that an adequate self-instructional set is established in the trainee, and that the trainee uses it appropriately in skill development.

Meichenbaum and Cameron (1973) have described a method for "teaching patients to talk to themselves" as a way to avoid distraction and guide performance in both familiar and unfamiliar tasks. Roder et al. (1988) suggest the following additional tactics to unburden working memory and facilitate functioning in the declarative stage of skill acquisition:

Use and Review Pertinent W-questions (What? Why?). Establishing the nature and purpose of a particular skill at the beginning is extremely important. Discussing why a certain skill should be practiced creates a meaningful context in which the individual is motivated to exert the mental effort to carry out an activity requiring use of the working memory. Without specific and directed effort, the patient may not establish such a context.

Begin with Simple Tasks. Training begun with a complex task may end in failure. This may so overload the working memory that a subsequent attempt, even at a less complex task, may seem meaningless to the patient. The load of a simple task is smaller and leaves working memory available for a subsequent task.

Adapt the Tempo and Allow for Breaks. The demand to work fast puts a further load on working memory, creating the risk of overload and task failure. Demands for faster performance can be introduced later, when skill automatization has reduced the load on working memory.

Execution of a task becomes automatic in the second stage of the learning process, *knowledge compilation*. As a task is successfully carried out a number of times with the aid of declarative information, the manner in which it is executed is stored in a program. This process is called *proceduralization*. After a skill has been proceduralized in a program, steps formerly guided by declarative self-instructions are linked together. This connection eliminates the need for step-by-step instructions, making capacity available in working memory and making it possible to execute the task faster. The linkage is called *composition*. Proceduralization and composition are achieved through repetition of the skill. Because of deficits in cognitive functioning, these processes are expected to occur more slowly in schizophrenic patients, requiring more repetitions for a given level of knowledge compilation. As with the declarative stage, a number of other training tactics serve to compensate for these difficulties:

Use and Review Pertinent W-questions (What? Which?). Posing W-questions is extremely important to proceduralization, specifically directing an action with questions such as "What are you going to do now?" and "Which step comes next?" Furthermore, patients must be taught to ask themselves these questions before and during the execution of a task.

Prompt. The posing of W-questions, as described here, may also be thought of as a form of prompting. When the prompt is given, the patient is to access information in working memory, which facilitates sequential performance of the skill components. More sequential repetition leads to more knowledge compilation and more available working memory capacity.

Use Self-talk as Feedback. In addition to serving as self-instructions, self-talk can be autoreinforcing. Giving oneself positive feedback when a job is well done increases motivation and further facilitates the process of knowledge compilation.

Proceed Step by Step through Training. In behavior therapy this technique is better known as shaping, a stepwise approach to a goal in which approximating steps are reinforced. Reinforcement of discrete steps in a task may compensate for the patient's difficulty in maintaining a motivational context for the task, at least long enough for relevant skills to be automatized, and for performance on the task to take on intrinsic or extrinsic reinforcing qualities.

In the third stage of the learning process, *production tuning,* learning is focused on the larger context in which the skill will be used. As there are many ways of carrying out a given task, context will determine the correct selection. Generalization and discrimination are key to this stage. Generalization brings about a gradual transition from task-specific skills to general skills with a greater range of application. Discrimination learning enables the person to identify those situations in which a specific skill is appropriate for performance.

It is well known that patients with schizophrenia, and to some degree other psychiatric patients, have great difficulty in appropriately performing new skills outside the context in which they were learned. A review of 114 studies of social skills training in various populations (Scott, Himadi, & Keane, 1984) estimated that although some degree of generalization is observed in 83 percent of the studies, less than 2 percent actually demonstrated new skill performance outside the training setting.

Failures in generalization have traditionally been explained in noncognitive terms. For example, the failures in social skills training are attributed to short training periods (trials of social skills training for schizophrenic patients are usually 10 to 20 hours of training), lack of specific training procedures to facilitate generalization, such as in vivo practice, and overemphasis on isolated skill components such as eye contact, voice volume, intonation, and body posture (Wallace et al., 1980). It has been estimated that if no attempt is made to practice skills outside therapy, the ability to demonstrate them at all will be lost within 6 to 12 months (Liberman, Massel et al., 1985; Liberman, Meuser et al., 1986). Conventional tactics for overcoming generalization and discrimination problems have therefore focused on more training, "booster" sessions, and training in varied settings.

In the production system model, generalization failures result from faulty or incomplete knowledge compilation. Environmental cues that would normally be signals to perform the skill are not included in the compilation, so those cues do not produce automatic task performance. Instead, cues peculiar to the training environment are compiled (for example, the trainer's verbal instructions), and only those cues develop automatic control over performance. Similarly, compilation of inappropriate cues limits discrimination. Such cues would normally indicate when a skill should be performed or inhibited, and in their absence skill performance occurs randomly.

The production system model thus generates at least two tactics for coping with generalization and discrimination problems not previously identified in conventional approaches:

Use Pertinent W-questions (When? What? Where? Who?). Selection of the correct cues for performing a skill is a condition for discrimination and generalization. Posing W-questions directed at specific cues is essential.

Include Explicit Training in Perception of Situations. Identification of cues must begin with attention and perception, which are often impaired in schizophrenic patients. Explicit training of attentional and/or perceptual skills may be necessary in such patients before they can include appropriate environmental information in their knowledge compilations.

Stress and Coping

Stress is generally recognized as an important factor in psychiatric disturbances (see Hinkle, 1974) and should therefore be considered in designing a rehabilitation program.

A number of investigators have established a link between stressful life events and the course of schizophrenia (for example, Brown & Birley, 1968; Brown, Birley & Wing, 1972; Sloof, 1984; Sanderman, 1988; Ventura et al., 1989). However, none of these studies established the precise relationship in time between life events and decompensation, or the predictive value of the events. Kanner et al. (1981) dispute the importance of major life events, emphasizing instead the role of "daily hassles," relatively small stresses that infringe upon the daily rhythm by causing irritation, frustration, or pain, and that demand a certain amount of adaptability. According to this theory, a life event could be the cause of a particular pattern of daily hassles. This pattern of hassles is the mediating factor between life events and psychopathology.

There has been no research on the quantitative relationship between daily hassles and schizophrenia. However, research on the relationship between expressed emotion (EE) and psychotic decompensation appears to be relevant. EE is a pattern of attitude and interpersonal communication, measured by observational scoring of communication samples obtained from relatives and others who know and interact with the patient. High EE is characterized by criticism, hostility, and emotional overinvolvement or overconcern directed at the patient. High EE creates an environment where many interpersonal daily hassles occur. It is well established that high EE increases the risk of psychotic relapse following discharge (Vaughn & Leff, 1976; Leff & Vaughn, 1985; Kuipers & Bebbington, 1988). Its predictive value is increased when EE is used in combination with other communication measures such as Communication Deviance (Singer & Wynne, 1966) and Affective Style (Doane et al., 1981).

The stress resulting from any particular life event is mediated by the subjective evaluation of the person under stress (Lazarus and Folkman, 1984). In other words, stress is in the eye of the beholder, and what is stressful to one person may not be so to the next. A number of intrapsychic factors may play a role in designating a life event as stressful, including locus of control, personality traits, and a person's general predisposition to fearfulness. For this reason, studies of daily hassles find that the sheer number of hassles a person experiences is independent of the level of stress subjectively reported (Reich, Parella & Filstead, 1988; Brantley et al., 1988). Similarly, the effects of stress are mediated by the person's actions consequent to the stressful event. The patterns of actions a person takes in response to stress are collectively termed coping.

Coping behavior is generally divided into *problem-oriented* versus *emotion-oriented*. In the first instance, the individual identifies the need for coping in response to a particular situation and then initiates appropriate behavioral strategies. In emotional coping, the person regards the problem as impossible to influence and takes self-protective measures. These are primarily fear-reducing measures such as avoidance, alcohol use, selective attention, reduced activity or acting-out behavior. Emotionally directed coping is typical in schizophrenic patients (Cohen & Berk, 1985) and may be seen as a means of preventing overstimulation. However, this manner of coping brings with it a new source of stress. Examples of schizophrenic emotional coping include social isolation (Cohen & Berk, 1985), seeking hospitalization (Lewis & Hugi, 1981), and deliberate stopping of medication with the intention of provoking a psychotic episode (Van Putten, Crumpton & Yale, 1976).

The coping concept gives the so-called negative symptoms another meaning. Many of these symptoms, such as social withdrawal, apathy, and lack of initiative, may be seen from this perspective as adaptation strategies. This calls for important changes in treatment. In the past these symptoms have been regarded as a form of psychopathology and treated as such. If this behavior is self-protective, then the goal of treatment should be learning a safe and socially acceptable alternative strategy, or learning problem-oriented coping. A number of symptoms, negative symptoms in particular, may then be seen as a form of coping behavior, developed as a reaction to vulnerability and to the course of schizophrenia.

Neuroleptic drugs (also known as antipsychotic drugs or major tranquilizers) have traditionally played a role in treatment of schizophrenia that conforms to the concepts of stress and coping. Neuroleptics facilitate coping by providing a biological buffer against stress. However, although drugs are now able to extend periods of remission, they cannot always prevent decompensation nor can they produce new coping skills (Hogarty et al., 1974). Neuroleptics are frequently necessary to facilitate skill acquisition. In that sense, they may be regarded as a necessary but incomplete "prosthetic" for skill acquisition.

GRIEF

Grief is a complex response pattern that follows a significant loss (Averill, 1968). Although such losses are always stressors, the nature of the grief response is such that coping responses may be less effective than when no loss is involved. Severe losses, such as death of a marital partner, can produce symptoms associated with severe psychiatric disorders, such as fatigue, memory problems, lack of interest, lack of concentration, restlessness, and even hallucinations (Clayton, 1990). Schizophrenic patients always experience important losses in self-efficacy, freedom and independence, and self-esteem. Some of these, such as losses in neuropsychological functions, may be permanent. Grief responses to these losses must be expected to influence the course of psychiatric rehabilitation. Grief is therefore a fourth central concept in program design.

Ramsay's (1977) grief model describes five stages in the grief process: shock, disorganization, denial, acceptance, and reintegration. The grief is resolved when it completes the last stage. Pathological grief can occur when the loss is denied or avoided. The natural grief process then becomes fixed in a specific stage, usually denial.

Behavior therapy supplies some important methods for facilitating the grief process (Kavanaugh, 1990). Grief therapies use the classical conditioning concept of *response extinction* to eliminate phobic avoidance of acknowledgment of the loss. Response extinction takes place through imaginal exposure of the patient to the details of the loss and its cognitive and emotional sequelae. Exposure leads the patient to experience that while the reality is difficult, it is manageable. As the grief process is being restarted through exposure, the patient's repertoire of cognitive and emotional coping skills is assessed and strengthened where indicated. Special techniques for coping with the depressive symptoms that usually accompany grief are also introduced.

Cognitive constructs related to the grief process can seriously hinder motivation for learning new skills. Constructs are logical structures that include assumptions and attributions, somewhat comparable to the popular notion of beliefs. Constructs are used not only to support and maintain static beliefs, but also to guide acquisition of new information and to revise continuously the ongoing interpretations of the world. In the language of Anderson's (1983) model, cognitive constructs exert an important influence on development and maintenance of production systems. In chronic psychiatric patients, such constructs are often associated with anticipation of failure, since all previous attempts at social integration have led to failure. When performance feedback is given in the course of rehabilitative skill training, it is important that the feedback not be processed through these constructs. The feedback must be presented by the therapist and processed by the patient in such a way that the inclination to cling to old, inefficient production systems is suppressed, while development of new production systems is fostered. This is facilitated by the following tactics:

Restructuring Learned Hopelessness. Irrational, habitual thoughts about failure and hopelessness continually interfere with rehabilitation progress. The therapist must be alert to this and must often assess actively, because patients may often experience such thoughts without verbalizing them. When detected, they should be addressed rationally by pointing out and giving examples of how the patient has strong and healthy parts, capable of controlling and overcoming handicaps.

Corrective Feedback. When the patient makes repeated mistakes, it may be because the therapist has not sufficiently divided the skill into meaningful steps. In that case, pointing out errors is superfluous. To optimize the training, corrective feedback should be used by the therapist as much as by the patient.

Positive Reinforcement. In Anderson's model, as well as in traditional behavior therapy, positive reinforcement is the most essential element in acquiring new skills and maintaining learned ones. Grief-related emotional reactions such as rebelliousness, aggression, extreme sadness, or feelings of hopelessness may interfere with the social process of positive reinforcement. It is important for the therapist (and others in the patient's environment) to identify these reactions as part of the grief process, rather than as undesirable characteristics of the patient that deserve criticism.

* * *

It is remarkable that so little attention has been paid in the psychiatric rehabilitation literature to systematic assessment and treatment of grief in schizophrenia. A possible reason is that research has traditionally been guided by "medical disease" models of the disorder. Such models usually focus attention on initial etiological processes, and they may neglect the long-term consequences of the acute disease process. The concept of psychiatric rehabilitation focuses instead on the disabilities and handicaps that result from the disease process. Reintegration of the person in the face of disabilities and handicaps is the goal of rehabilitation, and in that sense the goal of rehabilitation is comparable to the goal of grief resolution. This similarity would suggest that in the rehabilitation process the handicaps and disabilities that constitute a patient's losses should be systematically identified so as to assure that the grief response to these losses runs its course.

There is bound to be controversy about how to manage response to loss in schizophrenia and related disorders. For example, one view is that when patients are confronted with the handicaps resulting from schizophrenia, they tend to react with apathy and negative symptoms, reactions that hinder rehabilitation. Informing the patient that schizophrenia is accompanied by permanent handicaps may therefore undermine the patient's fundamental motivation for rehabilitation (Strauss et al., 1989). However, a grief process model would predict this reaction and would suggest a more confrontational approach to treatment based on exposure and development of coping skills.

The Concept of Rehabilitation

As the grief issue shows, the concept of rehabilitation itself introduces new perspectives that must be taken into account in the technological design of treatment programs. The aims of rehabilitation include the patient's acknowledgment of vulnerability to psychotic episodes, compensation for functional disturbances and handicaps through the development of adaptive or coping strategies, development of effective role behavior, and achievement of a gratifying position in the community (Watts & Bennet, 1983; Cnaan et al., 1988). These goals are not addressed in traditional medical treatment models, and the traditional concepts of cure and prevention take on secondary importance in rehabilitation. Cure is too elusive to be realistically expected, and prevention is intended only to ward off further deterioration and relapse. Optimal integration into the community and quality of life in a suitable living situation are the ultimate objectives of a rehabilitation program.

In traditional models, the purpose of diagnosis is to identify the etiology, and therefore the preferred treatment, of presenting symptoms. In rehabilitation, diagnosis is concerned primarily with identification of functional disturbances, ineffective coping strategies, social role limitations, and the supporting and limiting aspects of the symptoms. The individual's personality is diagnostically important, as it may hinder acceptance of handicaps. In the social environment, diagnosis serves to evaluate rejection reactions, interpersonal dependency, and stress factors such as the EE level.

Traditional treatment settings, most notably psychiatric wards, have a hospital-like atmosphere of orderly routines, hierarchical social structure, appointments, and rules. Implicit in long-term institutionalization is a high level of EE. In rehabilitation the hospital-like atmosphere is replaced by one of flexibility, accompanied by a low level of EE. An atmosphere of equality and responsibility for oneself should be fundamental in rehabilitation and residential wards. In other words, the living situation should be one in which patients can learn, using learning theory methods, to participate in the organization of the household and daily activities.

On traditional medical treatment wards, the patient is regarded as someone who is ill with a temporary disorder and needs protection and care, and whose symptoms must be treated. On traditional psychotherapy wards, the principle of constrained relationships is central; the goal is formation of a temporary dependency relationship, which is expected to develop into a harmony of independence and reciprocity. On rehabilitation wards, the patient is seen as a permanently vulnerable person, whose handicaps and symptoms must be recognized and accepted by everyone concerned. Therapy must be directed at optimizing the patient's social role functioning, including, as far as possible, self-reliance and independence in social relationships. The goal is to be achieved with individually adapted, possibly permanent, therapeutic support. On residential rehabilitation wards, the patient is regarded as a resident. The right to self-determination is primary. Attempts to achieve a low EE climate are based on the idea that what would not be tolerated in normal homes is not to be tolerated in the patient care setting.

On traditional treatment wards, the patient is someone who is sick, temporarily immature—not grown-up. On rehabilitation wards, the patient is a student. Rehabilitation patients have an important role in their treatment.

In traditional treatment, family members are thought of as possible factors in the etiology of the patient's disease or as passive secondary victims of the disease. On rehabilitation wards they are seen as influential and potentially supportive participants. Family members must themselves be well informed and supported so that they accept that the patient is handicapped, cannot be expected to respond to some normal demands, yet must accept as much personal responsibility as possible for optimal functioning and quality of life.

From a historical perspective, the most important impetus for the implementation of psychiatric rehabilitation is the fact that chronic psychiatric patients are nonproductive workers (Watts & Bennet, 1983). The first efforts at professional rehabilitation came about because of the need to reintegrate survivors of World War I into the workforce. Today the function of "work" is still a key to rehabilitation. Successful participation in meaningful work is essential for the development of independence, social valuation, self-appraisal, and social contact (Cnaan et al., 1988). Performance of the worker's role demands intact functioning at all levels of psychological organization—perceptual, attentional, cognitive, behavioral, and social. Thus doing some form of work enhances development of highly generalizable skills.

Schizophrenia has a particularly poor prognosis in the domain of returning to a functional worker role. Only about a third of patients find work following discharge, independent of whether they have had therapy explicitly directed at work performance (Anthony, Howell & Danley, 1984; Harding et al., 1987a). Half of these work at manual labor. Inclusion of some type of work therapy in a rehabilitation program for chronic schizophrenics will not guarantee that work skills and opportunities will be greater following discharge than before. However, this word of caution applies mainly to traditional work therapy, occupational therapy, or vocational rehabilitation. In psychiatric settings, these are often a sort of obligatory busy work, that patients are required to perform although it reflects neither their own motivation nor the skills they possess. The motivation for involvement may be primarily the staff's motivation to get the patient off the ward for a while. Traditional approaches fail to address the fact that in schizophrenia an important cause of the loss of a job is not an inability to do the work, but a lack of skills at the emotional and interpersonal level. Similarly, job-finding skills are often deficient in schizophrenic patients, so that even when they have appropriate vocational abilities they are unable to apply them in a community setting.

Work therapy in a rehabilitation program should be linked to individual patient needs and motivation and should be designed to create a meaningful context for rehabilitation and its goals. Training in social skills and job-finding skills occupies an important place in current rehabilitation therapy programs (Wallace et al., 1980).

A Comprehensive Rehabilitation Program

The theories and methods described above form the basis for a comprehensive rehabilitation program for individuals with chronic schizophrenia who have experienced long-term institutionalization. This program has as its goal the reversal of institutionalization by preparing patients for living either independently or in protected situations outside the clinic. Admission criteria for this program include a diagnosis of schizophrenia, at least five years' duration of illness, clinical picture consistent with institutionalization, and voluntary participation. Exclusion criteria include involuntary commitment or no voluntary participation in the program, demonstrated addiction, frequent self-mutilating behavior, and serious mental retardation. Potential participants who at the time of application are seriously psychotic are not refused but are placed in an intake unit where the acute psychosis is treated, primarily with medication. When the acute psychosis is controlled, the participant begins the program. The program is implemented in a 20-bed ward, 16 beds of which are allocated to the rehabilitation program and are divided between two groups of eight participants. Two of the remaining beds are for intakes. The rest are for use by patients ready to leave the program but for whom no protected living situation is available, or no other housing at all.

The eight-month rehabilitation program is divided into two four-month stages. The first stage is directed at learning to accept and deal with vulnerability and at developing basic skills. The second focuses on learning to deal with external sources of stress, optimizing self-care, seeking an appropriate residence, and developing daily activities. While the program is carried out in groups, the various training techniques are individualized as far as possible, so that, in principle, the participants follow the program at their own levels. Along with the program, each participant has a mentor—an attendant who acts as a personal supervisor and can, if necessary, also act as intermediary between the participant and family.

The comprehensive program is partially based on Integriertes Psychologisches Therapie-programm (Integrated Psychological Therapy Program, IPT), developed by Roder et al. (1988). IPT takes the form of formal group therapy sessions held several times each week. The program consists of three major divisions. The second and third divisions are very similar to programmed social and interpersonal skills training programs commonly found in American psychiatric rehabilitation. The first division focuses on more basic levels of functioning, such as concept formation and social perception. This unique feature until recently had no counterpart in American rehabilitation. The version described here (and in more detail in chap. 8 of this volume) amplifies the original version by combining group and individual sessions for development of specific cognitive abilities. Although various versions of IPT are in use throughout Europe, no study has yet shown that explicit training of cognitive functions is more effective than a conventional social skills program that lacks such explicit training. Investigation of the unique contribution of the cognitive component of IPT is the primary research mission of the rehabilitation program.

In addition to IPT, the program uses a number of less formal approaches derived from the theoretical principles discussed earlier in this chapter:

Psychoeducation of Participants. A willingness by clinicians to encourage and answer questions concerning the nature and course of a psychiatric illness and its emotional sequelae is a direct consequence of seeing patients as students and partners in treatment. If patients have an overview of their situation and the limitations of their possibilities, they can distance themselves from the patient role and develop other capabilities. Imparting information about schizophrenia is therefore central to the comprehensive program. This information includes discussion of symptoms, aftereffects, chronic factors, treatment, the social and legal consequences of a chronic psychosis and hospitalization, causes, and the various concepts of the vulnerability model. Additionally, grief-related processes such as aggression, jealousy, rebellion, despair, and hope—and in a broader sense, acceptance and self-esteem—are discussed. More routine human problems are also discussed, such as fear of failure, sexuality, and substance abuse. In addition to the obvious health education effects, psychoeducation provides therapeutic exposure as it does in cognitive-behavioral therapies for grief reactions, and therefore serves to reduce denial of handicaps or the risk of relapse.

Patient psychoeducation takes place in group meetings, usually with a nondirective discussion following more didactic presentation of information. The didactic part lasts no more than 20 minutes to avoid overstimulaton or fatigue.

Psychoeducation of the Family. The family also receives information about schizophrenia. Experience shows that in spite of support organizations for members of schizophrenic patients' family members (most notably in the United States, the Alliance for the Mentally Ill), many of them have been wrestling for years with the problems of their "sick" child or partner without ever having an opportunity to talk openly with members of other families and those in charge of treatment. Exchanging experiences and discussing ways to cope with the psychotic behavior of another is one of the main purposes of these sessions.

Weekly Evaluation. Current interpersonal problems are discussed during a weekly evaluation session. The depth of the discussion is determined by the group, guided by the group leader, with the aid of W-questions, toward solutions rather than the causes of individual or group dynamics. There is a danger of stimulating avoidance behavior when establishing what topics will be discussed; it is therefore very important to strive for agreement among participants about topic selection. This also requires close attention to the possible self-protective function of avoidance. Extremely restless or easily overstimulated participants may consciously avoid such sessions in order to prevent increased distress or decompensation.

Planning Days and Weekends; Agenda Training. Democratization and emancipation are important goals for the ward atmosphere. Staff must have the opportunity to demonstrate that they do not view the participants as sick people who need attention, but as equals, with a handicap, who must be conditioned to organize and lead their own lives. Rules may apply only when they have been established within a democratic decision-making structure where all present have an equal voice. During agenda training, all topics bearing on the program, management of the household, and organization of the ward are discussed, for example, division of household tasks and cooking duties, ward regulations and group activities.

Agenda training, conducted like a business meeting, is based on a permanent agenda. Activity planning is a stepwise approach to the central plan, using W-questions as a guideline. With regard to weekend planning, experience has shown that participants are inclined to become very passive over the weekend, often spending the whole time lying in bed. To address this problem, pre- and postweekend sessions are included in the program. Weekend planning is carried out in combination with the weekly evaluation. Evaluation of the weekend is done in two parts, a short, individual conversation and an evaluation as part of the agenda training. The purpose of the individual conversation is to discover what important unpleasant and pleasant events have taken place during the weekend. Central to the combined evaluation and agenda training is the evaluation of planning. When a plan is not carried out, the reason is discussed. When the problems are fundamental, clearly requiring more time than is available, they will be taken up during a weekly session with an individual therapist or during the weekly evaluation. When possible, the group explores successful ways for carrying out a plan that has failed.

Planning Free Time. Apathy and loss of initiative may result partially from an inability to plan free time. The planning and carrying out of group activities are a part of the training program. A stepwise approach to making a plan and the use of W-questions are essential for this.

News (Current Events) Orientation. Watching news programs on television daily is a permanent part of the program. The purpose is is to encourage community orientation. Moreover, talking about world events is a part of community orientation during the second stage.

Psychomotor Training. Body language, or nonverbal communication, is important for competent social interaction. However, tension and lack of control over arousal is common in schizophrenic patients, leading to deficits in psychomotor expression. Individual psychomotor training begins by teaching awareness of various muscle functions and proceeds by teaching techniques for relaxing. This phase of training ends with an opportunity to practice body language in social interaction.

Work Skills Training. The functions central to this training are attendance, cooperating with others, independence, staying power, tempo, distractibility, and concentration. This combination of cognitive functions is related to work skills and capabilities such as those often listed by employers in job advertisements. Participants decide together with the trainer which function they want to work on. In addition to optimizing functions, learning to accept one's limits and finding ways to perform a worker role in spite of these handicaps are essential. When a function is selected, a step-by-step plan is devised to implement a particular task. Assignments or projects are not the goal of training, but rather a means of developing work skills. After the first stage of training, the participants take an extensive career choice test. The results of this test determine the starting point for the second stage, which works toward developing a job or education.

A number of business and educational institutions cooperate with the program by allowing visits and by providing information about demands that employment or enrollment would create. With the help of staff, the patients evaluate themselves against these criteria to make vocational or educational decisions and to identify the skills they will need to pursue those plans.

Menu Planning and Cooking. Putting together a menu, planning the shopping, doing the shopping, and handling money are part of this training, as is learning to cook various menus. To this end a special cookbook that has been assembled describes and illustrates a number of dishes according to a step-by-step method.

Housekeeping Training. All household activities are taught. A text describing household tasks step by step is used.

Personal Care. Awareness of one's appearance and its effect on social interaction are important objectives of training in body and clothing care. An awareness of personal care and hygiene and healthy eating habits are developed with the help of a dietician and a beautician. This aspect of training also includes learning to make minor clothing repairs and to budget money, again according to a step-by-step plan.

Community Orientation. In this course various living situations are investigated and visited. A basic consideration is the required level of functioning with regard to arising, tidying the room, preparing a meal, daily activities, managing medication, social skills, and finances. Participants score their own levels of independence in these functions and compare the scores with the demands of a particular living situation. The score differences determine the starting point for training, with help from staff mentors. During this course specific attention is given to budgeting and to learning the rules governing various public resources, such as disability entitlement programs.

Physical Conditioning and Sports. Patients participate in aerobic fitness training such as that offered in every YMCA or YWCA or athletics club. In addition, all are encouraged to participate in sports organized by program staff.

Independent Housekeeping and Cooking. The participants do their own housekeeping on the ward and cook their own meals five times a week. This requires planning meals, shopping, and budgeting. Assistance is given only when indicated.

TENTATIVE RESULTS

At this time 45 patients have been admitted to the training program, 34 men and 11 women. The average age is 30.2 years. Participants experienced their first psychotic episode an average of 6.6 years before entering the program and had been hospitalized an average of 3.6 times before being transferred to the rehabilitation ward. The last hospitalization before referral lasted an average of 11.8 months. Twenty of the 45 participants are single, 6 have a permanent relationship, and 19 were living at home with their families prior to admission.

Five individuals (14 percent) left before finishing the program. All were men and all left within the first two months of the program. Three participants left because they felt they were "completely cured." Two of the three took up independent residence, and the third returned to his family. One participant left because he found the program too demanding. The last participant to leave early was rehospitalized for psychosis.

Among the 26 participants who have finished the program, 11 (42 percent) were referred to and accepted in a protected residential living situation, and 8 (30 percent) took up independent residence. For 7 participants (28 percent) some form of institutionalization was indicated following the program. Participants who are living independently have all found some form of daily activity, ranging from taking part in a paid workshop within the hospital to attending classes, and one paying job in the community. At this time none of these participants has been rehospitalized.

With regard to symptoms, skills, and general behavior, there is a clear tendency to improve from moment to moment. It is notable that this improvement is not stage-bound; improvement during the second stage of the program is not greater than during the first stage.

So far, the program appears to be effective in preventing institutionalization, suppressing symptoms, and developing skills and complex cognitive functions. The lack of any stage-specific effects may indicate that by integrating all relevant methods in all activities, the program creates a synergistic effect, wherein improvement in any one area facilitates improvements in other areas.

Concluding Comments

Developing a rehabilitation program such as the one described here is like setting up a schizophrenia school. Pupils are educated in coping with handicaps and developing skills. Much of the training is presented in the form of textbooks and other teaching procedures specially designed for the learning impediments characteristic of schizophrenia. The effects of taking cognitive impairments into consideration go beyond simple facilitation of skills acquisition, however. For example, the staff have observed that problems common in treatment of schizophrenia, such as running away, restlessness, and verbal confusion, either seldom occur or are more manageable when they do. It is interesting that although the program provides a fairly intensive schedule of activities, the rate of participation remains about 75 percent, rather high for schizophrenic patients. This is especially interesting in that the patients are not required to participate in any of the activities

The meaning of schizophrenia changes for both therapists and families when seen in the perspective of cognitive impairments and grief process theory. What was formerly attributed to lack of motivation comes to be seen as incapacity. This provides a new strategy for engaging the patient in treatment. One cannot change a person's motivation without changing that person's values and desires. One can treat cognitive and emotional impairments, however, and when such treatment is successful, motivation almost miraculously appears. This is congruent with the growing consensus among researchers, clinicians, and others that despite schizophrenic patients' notorious noncompliance with treatment, their values and aspirations are no different from anyone else's.

The central role that grief processing occupies in the program causes periods of depression and social withdrawal in many participants. During these periods problems of accepting disability become central. This development, although positive, has negative consequences for attending training and, in turn, a negative effect on rehabilitation progress. Maintaining the balance between rehabilitation progress, confrontation of disability, and avoidance of coercion becomes a difficult problem in clinical judgment.

Ward personnel and trainers feel tremendous pressure to rehabilitate the participants, who would otherwise be directly transferred to institutional wards. The sense of pressure can create a critical attitude toward the participants that might stand in the way of their achieving positive results for their efforts. To avoid this result, together with the unconventional methods used, personnel need to unlearn traditional methods and attitudes. Further education and ongoing supervision are required, perhaps more than in more traditional (and less effective) programs.

It is the basic assumption of the program that generalization of skills will improve through cognitive training and learning of coping strategies. Progress can be seriously hampered by the lack of an outpatient service network where learned skills are maintained and possibly broadened. Such a network is generally lacking in The Netherlands in spite of the fact that it has an extensive health care system compared with other countries (including the United States). Although the government is attempting to reduce the number of hospital beds and to create more protected living situations, at present there are limits on the residential care available for patients who have completed the rehabilitation program.

References

Anderson J. R. (1983). *The architecture of cognition.* Cambridge, Mass.: Harvard University Press.

Anthony, W. (1979). *The principles of psychiatric rehabilitation.* Amherst, Mass.: Human Resources Development Press.

Anthony, W. A., Howell J., & Danley K. (1984). The vocational rehabilitation of the psychiatrically disabled. In M. Mirabi (Ed.), *The chronically mentally ill: Research and practice*. New York: SP Medical And Scientific Books.

Averill, J. (1968). Grief: Its nature and significance. *Psychological Bulletin* 70, 721–748.

Bellack, A., Morrison, R., & Mueser, L. (1989). Social problem solving in schizophrenia. *Schizophrenia Bulletin,* 15, 101–116.

Benton, M. K., & Schroeder, H. E. (1990). Social skills training with schizophrenics: a meta-analytic evaluation. *Journal of Consulting and Clinical Psychology,* 58 (6), 741–747.

Brantley, P., Cocke, T., Jones, G., & Goreczny, A. (1988). The Daily Stress Inventory: Validity and effect of repeated administration. *Journal of Psychopathology & Behavior Assessment,* 10, 75–81.

Brown, G., & Birley, J. (1968). Crises and life changes and the onset of schizophrenia. *Journal of Health and Social Behavior,* 9, 203–214.

Brown, G., Birley, J., & Wing, J. (1972). Influence of family life on the course of schizophrenic disorders: A replication. *British Journal of Psychiatry,* 125, 121–258.

Clayton, P. (1990). Bereavement and depression. *Journal of Clinical Psychiatry,* 51(7), 34–38.

Cnaan, R., Blankertz, L., Messinger, K., & Gardner, J. (1988). Psychosocial rehabilitation: Toward a definition. *Psychosocial Rehabilitation Journal,* 11(4), 61–77.

Cohen, C., & Berk, L. (1985). Personal coping styles of schizophrenic outpatients. *Hospital and Community Psychiatry,* 36, 407–410.

Cowan, G., Conger, J., & Conger, A. (1989). Social competency and social perceptivity in self and others. *Journal of Psychopathology and Behavioral Assessment,* 11(2), 129–142.

Doane, J., West, K., Goldstein, M., Rodnick, E., & Jones, J. (1981). Parental communication deviance and affective style: Predictors of subsequent schizophrenia spectrum disorders in vulnerable adolescents. *Archives of General Psychiatry,* 38, 679–685.

Harding, C., Brooks, G., Ashikaga, T., Strauss, J., & Breier A. (1987a) The Vermont Longitudinal Study of Persons with Severe Mental Illness: Methodology, study sample and overall status 32 years later. *American Journal of Psychiatry,* 144(6), 718–726.

Harding, C., Brooks, G., Ashikaga, T., Strauss, J., & Breier A. (1987b). The Vermont Longitudinal Study of Persons with Severe Mental Illness: Long-term outcome of subjects who retrospectively met DSM-3 criteria for schizophrenia. *American Journal of Psychiatry,* 144(6), 727–735.

Hinkle, L. (1974). The concept of "stress" in the biological and social sciences. *International Journal of Psychiatric Medicine,* 5, 355–357.

Hogarty, G., Goldberg, S., Schooler, N., & Ulrich, R. (1974). Drug and sociotherapy in the aftercare of schizophrenic patients: II. Two year relapse rates. *Archives of General Psychiatry,* 31, 603–608.

Kanner, A., Coyne, J., Schaefer, C., & Lazarus, R. (1981). Comparison of two modes of stress measurement: Daily hassles and uplifts versus major life events. *Journal of Behavior Medicine,* 4, 1–39.

Kavanagh, D. (1990). Towards a cognitive-behavioral intervention for adult brief reactions. *British Journal of Psychiatry,* 157, 373–383.

Kuipers, L., & Bebbington, P. (1988). Expressed emotion research in schizophrenia: Theoretical and clinical implications. *Psychological Medicine,* 18, 893–909.

Lazarus, R., & Folkman, S. (1984). *Stress, appraisal and coping.* New York: Springer Publishing.

Leff, J., & Vaughn, C. (1985). *Expressed emotion in families: Its significance for mental illness.* New York: Guilford Press.

Lewis, D., & Hugi, R. (1981). Therapeutic stations and the chronic mentally ill. *Social Service Review,* 55, 206–220.

Liberman, R., Massel, H., Mosk, M., & Wong, S. (1985). Social skills training for chronic mental patients. *Hospital and Community Psychiatry,* 36(4), 396–403.

Liberman, R., Meuser, K., Wallace, C., Jacobs, H., Eckman, T., & Massel, H. (1986). Training skills in the psychiatrically disabled: Learning coping and competence. *Schizophrenia Bulletin,* 12(4), 631–647.

McGlashan, T. (1988). A selective review of recent North American long-term followup studies of schizophrenia. *Schizophrenia Bulletin,* 14(4), 515–542.

Meichenbaum, D., & Cameron, R. (1973). Training schizophrenics to talk to themselves: A means of developing self-controls. *Behavior Therapy,* 4, 515–534.

Ministerie van Welzijn, Volksgezondheid en Cultuur (1984). *Nota Geestelijke Volksgezondheid.* Gravenhage: Staatsuitgeverij.

Ramsay, R. (1977). Behavioral approaches to bereavement. *Behaviour Research & Therapy,* 15, 131–135.

Reich, W., Parrella, D., & Filstead, W. (1988). Unconfounding the Hassles Scale: External sources versus internal responses to stress. *Journal of Behavior Medicine,* 11, 239–249.

Roder, V., Brenner, H., Kienzle, N., & Hodel, B. (1988). *Integriertes Psychologisches Therapieprogramm fur schizophrene Patienten (IPT).* Munich: Psychologie Verlags Union.

Sanderman, R. (1988). *Life events, mediating variables and psychological distress: A longitudinal study.* Gröningen: Akademisch Proefschrift.

Scott, R., Himadi, W., & Keane, T. (1984). A review of generalization in social skills training: Suggestions for future research. *Progress in Behavior Modification,* 15, 113–172.

Singer, M., & Wynne, L. (1966). Principles for scoring communication defects and deviances in parents of schizophrenics: Rorschach and TAT scoring manuals. *Psychiatry,* 29, 260–288.

Slooff, C. (1984). *De klassifikatie en het beloop van schizofrene en reactieve psychosen*. Doctoral Dissertation, University of Gröningen.

Slooff, C. (1988). Het beloop en de afloop van schizofrene psychosen. In R. van den Bosch, C. van Meer, P. Dingemans & D. Linzen (Eds.), *Schizofrenie, recente ontwikkelingen in onderzoek en behandeling*. Deventer: Van Loghum Slaterus.

Strauss, J., Rakfeldt, J., Harding, C., & Liberman, R. (1989). Psychological and social aspects of negative symptoms. *British Journal of Psychiatry*, 155(7):128–132.

Stuurgroep Toekomstscenario's Gezondheidszorg (1990). *Zorgen voor Geestelijke gezondheid in de toekomst*. Utrecht: Bohn Scheltema & Holkema.

tenHorn, G. (1986). "Wat heet chronisch?" De GGZ-klienten van 1975, zes jaar later. *Provinciaal Register*, Afd. Sociale Psychiatrie Gröningen.

Van Putten, T., Crumpton, E., & Yale, C. (1976). Drug refusal and the wish to be crazy. *Archives of General Psychiatry*, 33, 1443–1446.

Vaughn, C., & Leff, J. (1976). The influence of family and social factors on the course of psychiatric illness. *British Journal of Psychiatry*, 129, 125–137.

Ventura, J., Nuechterlein, K., Lukoff, D., & Hardesty, J. (1989). A prospective study of stressful life events and schizophrenic relapse. *Journal of Abnormal Psychology*, 98(4), 407–411.

Wallace, C., Nelson, C., Liberman, R., Aitchison, R., Lukoff, D., Elder, J., & Ferris, C. (1980). A review and critique of social skills training with schizophrenic patients. *Schizophrenia Bulletin*, 6(1), 42–63.

Watts, F., & Bennett, D. (1983). *Theory and practice of psychiatric rehabilitation*. New York: Wiley.

Wing, J. (1978). *Schizophrenia: Towards a new synthesis*. London: Academic Press.

Zubin, J., & Spring, B. (1977). Vulnerability: A new view of schizophrenia. *Journal of Abnormal Psychology*, 86, 103–126.

• 8 •

Cognitive Training of Schizophrenic Patients: A Behavioral Approach Based on Experimental Psychopathology

M. van der Gaag, F. M. J. Woonings, R. J. van den Bosch, M. T. Appelo, C. J. Slooff, and J. W. Louwerens

This chapter describes the theory, practice, and outcome of a cognitive training program for schizophrenia. Originally developed as an innovative approach to treatment, the program is currently being implemented as a component of the comprehensive rehabilitation program described in chapter 7 of this volume.

Since the training program draws on a number of models of normal and abnormal cognition, key principles from those models will be reviewed first.

General Models of Cognition and Performance

Current models of human cognition distinguish between two general types of information processing: controlled and automatic (Shiffrin & Schneider, 1977). Automatic information processing is unconscious and very fast, and it is triggered by known and invariant stimuli. Several automatic processes can take place at the same time in a parallel way, since channel capacity is virtually unlimited. Generally learning has no influence on genetically programmed automatic perceptual processes, such as the encoding of spatial, temporal, and frequency information. Other automatic processes, sometimes called procedures, develop by practice and are important because they prevent overload of the processing system when complex skills, such as reading, dancing, driving a car, and the like, are being executed.

Controlled processing, on the other hand, is slow and proceeds in a step-by-step way. These processes are initiated and executed under supervisory control of conscious and voluntary attention. Controlled processes have a restricted capacity and they are vulnerable to overload and distraction. These processes require processing capacity for successful performance and they are characterized by the subjective experience as well as physiological signs of mental effort and fatigue. Controlled processing is required by much human behavior, in particular by tasks that need planning, choice making, reasoning, and problem solving. Controlled processing is also involved in skill acquisition and memory storage, for example, in the form of active rehearsal. Executive control is involved in selective attention, when decisions have to be made as to which stimuli should be selected for processing, and more generally in all kinds of strategic control of cognition.

The central executive function fulfills its task by controlling the activating mechanisms of the brain. Cognitive theories tend to emphasize computational mechanisms, but the functions of the brain are also controlled by arousal and activation. The arousal system is believed to control perception, while the activation system controls motor output (Tucker & Williamson, 1984; Pribram & McGuinness, 1975). The arousal system reacts to stimulus qualities. Novel and unexpected stimuli raise the level of arousal, resulting in a reduced reaction to known stimuli (habituation) and a greater response to novel and unexpected stimuli. This mechanism guarantees that the organism is alert to a changing environment, so that it can quickly adapt. Activation is involved in goal-directed action. The activation mechanism induces a lack of interest in momentary stimuli, and it motivates the organism to aim for rewarding goals in the future. Disruption of ongoing behavior requires an emotional (arousal) response. Inhibition of distraction by novel stimuli and motivated action need activation. Both arousal and activation are coordinated by a control mechanism associated with the phenomenological experience of "effort."

It is generally assumed that schizophrenia is characterized by relatively intact automatic processes but that controlled processes tend to be dysfunctional. This failure in controlled information processing is associated with activation dysfunctions, and it has important consequences for the learning of skills. Skills develop by automatization as they are practiced. For instance, learning to drive a car is a controlled process at the outset. A student driver has to instruct himself consciously while driving, and many errors characterize this stage. With practice a skill is gradually compiled into a procedure (Anderson, 1983). The acquisition of new skills involves a gradual transition from declarative, conscious knowledge into procedural, preattentive ("automatic") knowledge. This transition includes a number of stages.

At the first stage, the subject uses declarative knowledge to guide behavior during task performance. The declarative stage puts a heavy load on working memory and effort. The subject, who experiences mental fatigue, is not able to perform a second task at the same time. After compilation, declarative knowledge is no longer required, the demands on working memory are reduced, and the speed of performance increases. The subject experiences less mental fatigue and finally it becomes possible to simultaneously perform a second task, e.g., talking to a passenger while driving. Once a skill has been compiled into a procedure, the learning process proceeds into the stage of production tuning. Within this stage a gradual continued improvement in performance can be observed, and it is characterized as a gradual transfer into skilled expertise.

Three learning principles can be distinguished. The generalization process accomplishes a gradual transfer from task-specific skills into more general skills that are applicable in various tasks. The discrimination process results in detailed knowledge about when to do what. Strengthening, or reinforcement, results in a hierarchical structure in procedural memory by facilitating the application of those skills that are most likely to be sucessful. It follows that schizophrenic patients who have problems with controlled processes will also have problems in acquiring skills, in the generalization of skills, and in refining skills by progressive discrimination learning. Rehabilitation programs should pay attention to these problems.

Cognitive Deficits and Psychotic Symptoms

Even during periods of remission, many schizophrenic patients experience difficulty with attention and memory. Acute psychosis deranges the organization of thought, but these phenomena are mostly transient. Cognitive deficits, therefore, are partly state-like and partly trait-like. Yet not all schizophrenic patients have cognitive deficits, whether subjectively experienced or measured by cognitive tasks. Some patients with florid hallucinations and delusions, in the absence of disorganization and psychomotor poverty, tend to have normal cognitive profiles (Liddle, 1987b, 1991; Bilder, 1985). We therefore have to assume that not all psychotic symptoms are direct manifestations of cognitive deficits, since some psychotic patients do not have these deficits. Models that propose that symptoms and behavior problems invariably arise from cognitive deficits can have only partial validity. Generally, trait-like cognitive deficits are differently associated with negative symptoms (apathy, flat affect, and the like), social deficit syndromes, and positive symptoms (such as delusions and hallucinations).

Wagman et al. (1987) examined neuropsychological function in 15 deficit and 15 matched nondeficit syndrome schizophrenics. Both schizophrenic groups performed poorly on a psychomotor measure, compared to normals. Only the deficit group performed worse on a general performance factor. The authors suggested that the poor performance of the deficit group might not be related to intellectual impairment, but to a subtle, global motivational impairment. The results were not associated with severity of either positive or negative symptoms at the time of testing.

Kolakowska et al. (1985) examined 65 patients (42 schizophrenia and 14 schizoaffective disorder) and found that performance on several cognitive tests tended to be lower in the poor- than in the good-outcome group, in inpatients with an unsatisfactory response to neuroleptics compared with responders, and in those with negative symptoms compared with other patients. Only conceptual impairment was related to positive symptoms, and both conceptual and verbal memory deficits were associated with negative symptoms. However, when the asymptomatic good-outcome group was disregarded and the analysis was limited to patients with poor and intermediate outcome, deficits in cognitive functions showed no association with clinical features within that sample. It is noteworthy that of the 15 subjects who showed both neurodysfunction and cognitive impairment, six had good outcome and seven had intermediate outcome. In contrast to the neurological abnormalities, cognitive impairment was related to the severity of the residual disorder. As expected, it was most pronounced in the poor-outcome group—patients with the most severe symptoms, behavior disorder, social deterioration, and resistance to treatment. Deficits in particular cognitive domains, but not general impairment, appeared to be related to positive and negative symptoms. The lack of association between neuropsychological deficit and the duration of illness is consistent with the findings of others (Goldstein & Zubin, 1990; Klonoff et al., 1970; Smith, 1964; Waddington, 1990).

An association between negative symptoms and cognitive deficits has also been found by other investigators. Green & Walker (1984) found negative symptoms to be associated with "slower information processing" in a backward making task. Kay et al. (1986) found negative symptoms to be correlated with deficits in cognitive, affective, social, and motor spheres, with a higher incidence of major psychiatric illness but less affective disorder among relatives, with lower education, and with greater cognitive developmental impairment. Cornblatt et al. (1985) used an information overload task and concluded that positive symptoms were related to distractibility, whereas negative symptoms were associated with lowered processing capacity. Whereas Kolakowska et al. (1985) found negative symptoms to be related to verbal memory, Green & Walker (1985) found that short-term verbal memory was related to positive symptoms. The latter investigators used the Token test and sentence repetition as measures, so what they called verbal memory might rather be called verbal comprehension. If so, positive symptoms, e.g., disorganization, could be responsible for these findings.

Addington et al. (1991) found negative symptoms to be related with general IQ, Word Fluency, and the error score on the Wisconsin Card Sorting Test (WCST). Visual spatial deficits were related to bizarre behavior. They retested their patients after six months, when they were in remission. Some tests improved, but deficits on Rey copy, WCST, Word Fluency, and delayed verbal memory persisted. Improvement was due to improvement in positive symptoms rather than to improvement in negative symptoms, although hallucinations were not related to cognitive deficits. Schmand (1991) found no relation between positive or negative symptoms and cognitive deficits on Continuous Performance Test, verbal memory (Rey), and Span of Apprehension. He did find an association between negative symptoms and energetical problems. A time-on-task effect (increase of reaction time during a simple task) was related to negative symptoms, vigilance, and verbal memory, but not to sensory storage. He concluded that cognitive disorders in psychotic patients can be explained better by activation deficits than by clinical symptoms.

Bilder et al. (1985) factor-analyzed symptoms and found three factors identical to those found by Liddle (1987a, 1987b, 1990, 1991) and Arndt et al. (1991). One cluster of symptoms (inadequate affect, thought disorder, and bizarre behavior) appeared to reflect primarily a disorganization of thought, independent of a negative factor (affective flattening, avolition/apathy, and anhedonia) and a positive factor (delusions, hallucinations). This disorganization factor was associated with language and memory deficits. The positive factor, when separated from thought disorder, was no longer associated with cognitive deficits. The negative factor, called psychomotor poverty by Liddle, had only a mild association with cognitive deficits.

These data taken together lead to the following picture:

1. Psychomotor poverty is associated with cognitive deficits characterized by diminished processing speed and reduced processing capacity;
2. Disorganization is associated with cognitive deficits characterized by distractibility, visuospatial/visuomotor dysfunctions and planning problems;
3. Reality distortion (delusions and hallucinations) is not associated with cognitive disorder;
4. A poor outcome is associated with duration of illness, but cognitive deficits have no association with duration of illness.

So disorganization is most disrupting to cognitive processing. This result points to problems in the organization of the processes, rather than to deficits in discrete stages of processing. In other words, consciously controlled and effortful processing seems to be disturbed in schizophrenics and automatic processing is largely undisturbed.

Schizophrenia Disrupts Controlled Processing

To prevent interference by incoming sensory information, the optimum level of arousal is low for controlled processes. If the level of arousal is too high, the reduced attentional capacity will lead to deficits on tasks that require controlled processing, such as memory tasks requiring active rehearsal and other mnemonic activities (Hasher & Zacks, 1979). So, the arousal regulation problems found in schizophrenic patients are likely to disturb controlled information processing predominantly. Callaway & Naghdi (1982) found automatic processes to be normal to hypernormal in schizophrenic patients.

Patients don't fall off their bicycles because of schizophrenia. This may sound obvious, but, from an information-processing point of view, it is important. To keep balance on a bicycle, very fast processing of multiple proprioceptive stimuli and vestibular information is needed. Although defense computers can calculate the interception point with incoming missiles at an incredible speed, these computers still are not fast enough to ride a bicycle.

We start walking when we are about one year of age and we can do this without experiencing mental effort. Yet the needed calculation capacity exceeds the capacity for playing chess. Schizophrenic patients have normal automatic processes in comparison with most neurological patients. Most patients can swim, dance the foxtrot, ride a bicycle, and play table tennis as we do, even when medicated. However, even schizophrenic patients who play excellent chess often lose a game because of a mistake made during a lapse in attention. Likewise, many other controlled processes, such as having a conversation, making a shopping list, cleaning and organizing a room, often cannot be accomplished by schizophrenic patients.

Controlled processes are easily disturbed because they have a flexible organization, involving most of the brain. Automatic processes are unconscious and subcortical, and the important neural pathways are those connecting the sensory areas with motor areas. Only controlled processes are open to training, because of their conscious nature. Some studies have provided evidence of improvement to normal levels after training in schizophrenic patients (e.g., Koh, Kayton & Peterson, 1976; Meiselman, 1970; Wagner, 1968). Callaway and Naghdi (1982) commented on the plasticity of these processes: "[they] are characteristically flexible, adaptive, and responsive to training; in schizophrenics, they can also be normalized with practice and improved by adequate experimenter-engineered motivation. . . . We suspect schizophrenics can adopt strategies that put more or less reliance on them" (p. 344).

One of the problems of the automatic versus controlled dichotomy is that there is no clear boundary between the two types. In fact this distinction is of a dimensional nature. Processes are more or less automatized and more or less controlled (Hasher & Zacks, 1979; Cohen et al., 1990). Controlled processes are also more or less effortful. The distinction is further blurred because controlled processes use automatized subroutines. These demarcational problems notwithstanding, it is clear that schizophrenic patients are suffering primarily from controlled processing deficits, and that this may result from, as well as create, activation problems.

ACTIVATION OF COGNITION IN SCHIZOPHRENIA

Activation dysfunctions in schizophrenia take several forms. Problems arising from overarousal are well-known. In normal circumstances overarousal is the result of overstimulation by high-intensity sensory input. Moderately high stimulus intensities give rise to an orienting response. When the stimulus is too intense, a defensive response will be the result. This response aims to reduce the painful or disorganizing influence of the stimulus. Consequences of overarousal on information processing are:

— Less attention for visual stimuli in the periphery (Korchin, 1964; Easterbrook, 1959);
— A perceptual bias toward very salient details (Schwartz, 1975) and a decreased discrimination between relevant and irrelevant stimuli (Broadbent, 1971);
— Less "deep" information processing (Schwartz, 1975; Craick & Lockhart, 1972)—that is, the processing of physical characteristics tends to dominate over the processing of semantic characteristics;
— A slowing down of the retrieval of information (Eysenck, 1975) and limiting the search to more accessible sources of knowledge (Eysenck, 1976);
— A switch from parallel processing to serial modes of processing (Wally & Weiden, 1973);
— More interference on tasks like the Stroop (Glass & Singer, 1972).

Gjerde (1983) has argued that much of schizophrenic performance deficits, symptoms, and behavior can be understood as the result of chronic overarousal. Depue (1974), for instance, found no differences between schizophrenics and a highly aroused group of normal controls.

Underarousal has not been the target of much information-processing research in schizophrenia. Underarousal will result in distractibility and failure to habituate. Arousal reduces the number of stimuli to be registered, by habituation of responses to stimuli that are not novel. Underaroused patients therefore tend to overreact to stimuli.

Overactivation is often the result of overarousal. Sanders (1983) described how overarousal, when not tuned down by effort, will result in immediate response, without conscious consideration. This type of behavior is characterized by rigid and stereotyped responding. Mistakes are not corrected and perseveration may occur.

Underactivation is most characteristic of the psychomotor poverty syndrome. Whereas faulty responding is characteristic of the state of overactivation, underactivation is characterized by lack of response. The corresponding symptomatology consists of poverty of speech, loss of initiative, flattening of affect, and the like.

Self-Protective Mechanisms

Broen (1973) has suggested that restricted perception could serve a defensive function. This strategy reduces the number of perceived relevant cues but pays off in the form of reduced distractibility. Silverman (1972) also argued that restricted monitoring should be considered a defensive style. Many schizophrenic patients show fewer orientation reactions, prefer low-complex stimuli over high-complex stimuli, and profit from sensory deprivation by reducing perceptual aberrations, whereas normals show an opposite reaction when deprived. Feeney (1971) found that a group of chronic nonparanoid schizophrenics had more difficulty detecting a signal that could be presented in two modalities (light or sound) than did either acute schizophrenics or normals. The chronic group restricted monitoring to one sensory modality. Her prediction—that the chronic group would be more distracted within the same modality than across modalities—was verified. If the distracting stimuli were presented in a different sensory modality, the chronic group was even less distracted than the acute group and performed as well as the normal controls. If the distracting stimuli were presented within the same modality, then both schizophrenic groups were more distracted than normals.

Broen suggested that considering the individual differences in distractibility among chronic schizophrenics, a number of chronic patients might persist in a restricted monitoring strategy even after they have recovered cognitively. In this subgroup, training should lead to more elaborate perceptual processing. The group with increased levels of distractibility would suffer from overstimulation during training and would be expected to persist in a restricted monitoring strategy.

The basic problem in schizophrenia does not seem to be a breakdown of parts of the information-processing apparatus, but a dysfunction of activating mechanisms. Arousal is a dynamic process that is optimized by feedback. In schizophrenic patients, central supervising systems seem unable to optimize the level of arousal to fit task demands, leading to problems with input regulation. This, in turn, provokes self-protective mechanisms aimed at preventing overload experiences. Miller (1960) has delineated a number of these adjustment processes aimed at reducing the subjective experience of information overload. These processes are:

1. Omission: temporary nonprocessing of information.
2. Error: processing of incorrect information.
3. Queuing: delaying the response in the hope that it will be possible to catch up later.
4. Filtering: neglecting to process certain categories of information.
5. Cutting categories: responding with less than optimum precision.
6. Employing multiple channels: processing information through several channels simultaneously.
7. Escape from the task.

Any clinician who is acquainted with schizophrenia will recognize the coping strategies of patients in handling everyday life situations in these processes, with the possible exception of employment of multiple channels. Omission, for instance, is a characteristic of schizophrenic performance on vigilance tasks like the Continuous Performance Test, but it can also be recognized in underresponsiveness and poverty of speech. Erroneous processing, often seen in schizophrenia, may be the result of filtering and cutting categories. Queuing can be recognized in long latencies before responding and in irregular performance on speed tasks. Filtering is caused by overarousal, which results in processing only part of the information available. It can also be a defensive strategy on a more conscious level and is then characterized by restricted processing. Cutting categories may also be interpreted as defensive processing. In fact, many patients use crude categories to oversimplify the world, thus relieving strain on processing resources. Many schizophrenic patients also tend to escape from tasks.

Starting Points for Cognitive Training

It is useful to distinguish between primary and secondary cognitive deficits. Primary cognitive deficits are stable, whereas secondary deficits are of a more transient nature. Many patients stick to a secondary, restricted, self-protective processing strategy even when it is no longer adequate. It is in these patients that cognitive training, as a kind of exposure treatment, can help to reestablish a more elaborated style of processing. This working hypothesis can explain the results of Brenner et al. (1980) and Olbrich & Mussgay (1990), who found improvement in performance on complex tests after cognitive training, while tests that measure more basic aspects of information processing were not affected.

Treatment of secondary deficits thus requires a cognitive training program that stresses elaborate processing of perceptual data by improving executive control. Memorizing, ordering, and planning should also be part of this training program, but to a lesser extent and in the service of social and interpersonal perception. Disturbing and distracting stimuli, like emotions, should be gradually introduced to desensitize the subjects and to enable them to keep arousal within limits that allow for adequate processing.

The cognitive deficits of schizophrenic patients disrupt the understanding of social situations. Emotion displayed in facial expressions or tone of voice—the context—is often wrongly interpreted. This also explains the disappointing experiences with social skills training in chronic patients having many negative symptoms. Skills training presumes that information can be processed smoothly and that it is only the skill that is lacking or inhibited. In fact, social skills are not lacking, since most patients have applied these skills before their psychotic breakdown. It is perception of the social environment that is disturbed and that causes skills to be elicited no longer at the right moment. When patients watch role-plays during social skills assessments, they often attend to irrelevant stimuli, like what the players are wearing, or to their own emotional responses. It is thus necessary to start rehabilitation by modifying the perceptual processes of these patients. Training should begin at a descriptive and matter-of-fact level, and then ascend to the perception and understanding of entire social situations, including the context in which emotions are to be understood and experienced.

General Strategies for Cognitive Training

The cognitive training programs developed at the Oegstgeest and Assen psychiatric hospitals uses components of the "cognitive differentiation" treatment developed by Brenner and his associates (1980). The Brenner approach utilizes group exercises and activities to strengthen attention, conceptual processing, memory, and social perception. The exercises range from attending to and simply repeating sentences read by other group members to telling and summarizing entire stories.

The Oegstgeest-Assen approach adds three main strategies to the Brenner exercises: an attention-focusing and planning strategy, borrowed from Meichenbaum & Cameron (1973); a mnemonic strategy, aiming at organizing the material during acquisition; and an analytical inductive reasoning strategy as a cognitive-behavioral prosthesis for failing perceptual processing of complex and emotional stimuli. The first and the second strategy are spontaneously applied by normal subjects but are deficient or lacking in schizophrenic patients. The third strategy is not typically used by normals, so it is artificial, of a prosthetic nature. All strategies aim to enforce what is called executive function or evaluation of performance.

THE SELF-INSTRUCTION ATTENTIONAL STRATEGY

The patient is told that behavior needs guidance in time-consuming or complex tasks. Constructive thoughts and considerations must be applied in the form of self-instructions. A set of five self-instructions is first rehearsed aloud, becoming more covert in later stages. Borrowed from Meichenbaum & Cameron, they are:

1. Questions about the demands of the task: "What is the goal of this task?" "What am I expected to accomplish?"
2. Step-by-step planning in advance: "First I should do this, then that, and I should not attend to . . ."
3. Self-instructions during task execution.
4. Self-talk as a coping strategy to handle faults and frustration: "This is a mistake, but let me see, I can correct it in this way." "When I keep quiet, I can do it."
5. Self-reinforcement during and after task performance: "This way it goes fine, I'm halfway now"; "I did this fine."

THE MNEMONIC STRATEGY

The patient is told that in order to remember, it is important to be active during acquisition. The following methods can be helpful:

1. to name aloud and rehearse several times,
2. to categorize the material, e.g., pleasant-unpleasant, small-big, red-blue,
3. to visualize the material in an image containing all stimuli,
4. to use memory aids, e.g. by making an easily remembered word of the first letters of each item to be remembered.

THE INDUCTIVE REASONING STRATEGY

Failing perception of complex social and emotional stimuli makes schizophrenic patients rely on a trial-and-error strategy. Patients often reach a premature, inadequate opinion based on only part of the information available; as a remedy, their analytical strategy is elaborated and refined. The patient is told to scan situations at ease and come to an interpretation by following a four-step process:

1. Give a matter-of-fact description of objects and persons: shape, color, clothing, and so on;
2. Characterize the actions of each person involved;
3. Form propositions about roles, motives, relations, and feelings, and check them against what can be perceived;
4. Characterize the theme of what is going on.

This ascension from sensory data to abstract meaning is also applied in the social perception parts of the Brenner rehabilitation program. A new element is an analytical procedure in the judgment of facial emotion. Patients are told which discrete features differentiate between emotions, so they do not have to globally assess the complete facial expression. The training itself is structured in such a way that optimum learning takes place. Verbal instructions are given sparsely. Modeling is used all the time. Complex skills are shaped over sessions and only reinforcement is given. Suggestions are made only after reinforcing the component skills. Patients are never criticized. Each exercise starts from the level of mastery and is then extended to more difficult levels. In addition to optimizing information processing, these procedures sustain motivation to engage in the tasks.

Evaluation of Treatment Outcome

A systematic evaluation of the effectiveness of the Oegstgeest-Assen program has been conducted. Preliminary results are described here. Full details are published in the doctoral dissertation of the first author (van der Gaag, 1992).

Five groups of subjects were examined. Two groups of schizophrenic inpatients were at the core of the experimental design: a group receiving cognitive training ($N = 21$) and an attention-placebo group ($N = 21$). The training program comprised 23 sessions and a total of 45 different exercises and included homework. There were three control groups: schizophrenic outpatients, affectively disordered outpatients, and normal controls. Diagnoses were made by a senior psychiatrist and a trainee in psychiatry according to the DSM-III-R criteria. All schizophrenic patient groups were matched on duration of illness. The training and the attention-placebo groups were matched on daily dosage of antipsychotic medication, age, level of education, and sex. Neuropsychological and cognitive measures were obtained before and after cognitive training. The following dependent measures were included:

Attention:
- Continuous Performance Test (Rosvold et al., 1956)
- Span of Apprehension Test (Estes & Taylor, 1966)
- Trail Making Test B (Halstead, 1947)
- Stroop Color-Word Test (Stroop, 1935)

Perception:
- Emotion Matching Test (van der Gaag & Haenen, 1990)
- Emotion Labelling Test (van der Gaag & Haenen, 1990)
- WAIS Picture Arrangement (Wechsler, 1958)
- GIT Visual Closure Test (Luteijn & Van der Ploeg, 1983)

Memory:
- Rey Auditory-Learning Test (Rey, 1964)
- Rey Complex Figure (Rey, 1964)
- WAIS Digit Symbol (Wechsler, 1958)
- GIT Word Fluency (Luteijn & Van der Ploeg, 1983)

Planning and reasoning:
- WISC Mazes (Dutch version, de Bruyn et al., 1986)
- Wisconsin Card Sorting Test (Berg, 1948; Nelson, 1976)

There was no improvement in either group on six measures: Continuous Performance, Span of Apprehension, Trail Making B, WAIS Digit Symbol, WISC Mazes, and GIT Word Fluency. There was equal improvement in both groups on three measures: Stroop Color-Word Test, GIT Visual Closure, and Rey Auditory-Learning. Training did not affect the scores on these tests. Improvements in the attention-placebo group are probably due to learning over trials, or test-retest effects. The Continuous Performance Test is a known vulnerability marker, so changes were not expected. WISC Mazes, Trail Making B, WAIS Digit Symbol, Span of Apprehension, and the Stroop Test are speed tests, as the raw scores are based on time to accomplish the task. So the conclusion has to be that speed (or efficacy) of information processing does not seem to be influenced by training. Word Fluency and Visual Closure are preattentive automatic tasks that are not open to cognitive mediation or cognitive strategies. Word Fluency performance gives no indication of how the searching process in memory is done. When a word pops up, one does not know how and where it was found. The same is true for Visual Closure. Either the drawing is recognized, or it is not.

Improvement occurred in the training group only on six measures: Emotion Matching Test, Emotion Labelling Test, Picture Arrangement, WCST, Rey Complex Figure, and Rey Auditory-Learning. In these tests, speed of processing is not important. It is accuracy that is measured, and there is no time pressure. These tasks are also open to a verbal-cognitive processing strategy. Both long-term memory tasks seem to have profited from the application of mnemonic strategies. The emotion tasks that could not be done appropriately before training because of failing global perception also benefited from training. The training apparently succeeded in replacing the failing global strategy by an inductive-reasoning strategy. Patients were taught which discrete features discriminated between different emotions. They seem to have learned how to apply rules from declarative memory. Performance on the Picture Arrangement task has probably benefited from this very inductive-reasoning strategy by scrutinizing details, appointing actions, and then proceeding with interpersonal relations, feelings, and motives.

Discussion

Initial development of the cognitive training program was based on a fairly simple model. Cognitive disturbances were assumed to be fundamental to symptoms and behavioral disorder. Facts turned out to be more complex. Not all schizophrenic patients have cognitive deficits, and therefore symptoms and behavioral deficits cannot be explained simply as a direct result of information-processing deficits. This implies that improvement of cognitive functioning is not likely to result automatically in clinical improvement and behavior change.

Cognitive deficits were not found to be correlated with duration of illness. Transient deficits can be present at any moment. Persisting and stable deficits are thought to be present before the first psychotic breakdown. The primary deficits are probably processing parameters such as efficacy of processing and capacity of processing. Training does not seem to improve these parameters. More complex processing, requiring mental effort, did improve. Deficits in this area are of a secondary nature and are probably due to an organizational defense against the threat of information overload that results from overarousal and disorganization. Some patients seem to stick to the self-protective strategy of restricted processing, giving up executive control, even when this is no longer necessary. These processes can be reestablished by training, which has the character of exercising cognitive processes and faculties to handle the natural flow of information from everyday life. It is quite possible that the effects of cognitive training are caused by desensitization or exposure rather than by a specific improvement of target functions.

There is no doubt that training cognitive functions is clinically relevant, since the measures that improved always reached levels typically found in outpatients and sometimes even normal levels. Although improved cognitive functioning does not directly result in improved symptom status or behavior change, it is a prerequisite for the effective learning of social skills. The patient with severe schizophrenic deficits is like a collapsed house of cards. One cannot start at the roof, but rebuilding the basement, on the other hand, does not imply that the other floors will be put in place automatically. After cognitive functioning improves, effective training of domestic and social skills becomes possible.

References

Addington, J., Addington, D., & Maticka-Tyndale, E. (1991). Cognitive functioning and positive and negative symptoms in schizophrenia. *Schizophrenia Research, 5*, 123–134.

American Psychiatric Association (1987). Diagnostic and statistical manual of mental disorders (3rd Ed., Rev.). Washington, D.C.: American Psychiatric Press.

Anderson, J. R. (1983). The architecture of cognition. Cambridge, Mass.: Harvard University Press.

Arndt, S., Alliger, R. J., & Andreasen, N. C. (1991). The distinction of positive and negative symptoms: The failure of a two-dimensional model. *British Journal of Psychiatry*, 158, 317–322.

Berg, E. A. (1948). A simple objective test for measuring flexibility in thinking. *Journal of General Psychology*, 39, 15–22.

Bilder, R. M., Mukherjee, S., Rieder, R. O., & Pandurangie, A. K. (1985). Symptomatic and neuropsychological components of defect states. *Schizophrenia Bulletin*, 11(3), 409–419.

Brenner, H. D., Stramke, W. G., Mewes, J., Liese, F., & Seeger, G. (1980). Erfahrungen mit einem spezifischen Therapieprogramm zum Training kognitiver und kommunikativer Fähigkeiten in der Rehabilitation chronisch schizophrener Patienten. Nervenarzt, 51, 106–112.

Broadbent, D. E. (1971). *Decision and stress*. New York: Academic Press.

Broen, W. E. (1973). Limiting the flood of stimulation: A protective deficit in chronic schizophrenia. In R. L. Solso (Ed.), *Contemporary issues in cognitive psychology*. Washington D. C.: Winston.

Callaway, E., & Naghdi, S. (1982). An information processing model for schizophrenia. *Archives of General Psychiatry*, 39, 339–347.

Cohen, J. C., Dunbar, K., & McClelland, J. L. (1990). On the control of automatic processes: A parallel distributed processing account of the Stroop effect. *Psychological Review*, 97(3), 332–361.

Cornblatt, B. A., Lenzenweger, M. F., Dworkin, R. H., & Erlenmeyer-Kimling, L. (1985). Positive and negative schizophrenic symptoms, attention, and information processing. *Schizophrenia Bulletin*, 11, 3, 397–407.

Craik, F. I., & Lockhart, R. S. (1972). Levels of processing: A framework for memory research. *Journal of Verbal Learning and Verbal Behavior*, 11, 671–684.

de Bruyn, E. E. J., van Haassen, P. P., Poortinga, Y. H., & Lutje Spelberg, H. C. (1986). Wechsler Intelligence Scale for Children. Revised; Dutch translation. Lisse, The Netherlands: Swets & Zeitlinger.

Depue, R. A. (1974). The specificity of response interference to schizophrenia. *Journal of Abnormal Psychology*, 83, 529–532.

Easterbrook, J. A. (1959). The effect of emotion on cue utilization and the organization of behavior. *Psychological Review*, 48, 177–203.

Estes, W. K., & Taylor, H. A. (1966). Visual detection in relation to display size and redundancy of critical elements. *Perceptual Psychophysics*, 1, 9–16.

Eysenck, M. W. (1975). Extraversion, arousal and speed of retrieval from secondary storage. *Journal of Personality*, 43, 390–391.

Eysenck, M. W. (1976). Arousal, learning and memory. *Psychological Bulletin*, 83, 389–404.

Feeney, S. (1971). Breadth of cue utilization and ability to attend selectively in schizophrenics and normals. Unpublished doctoral dissertation, University of California, Los Angeles.

van der Gaag, M. (1992). *The results of cognitive training in schizophrenic patients*. Delft, The Netherlands: Eburon.

van der Gaag, M., & Haenen, M. A. (1990). Schizophrenia and the impaired evaluation of facial affect. In P. D. J. Drenth et al. (Eds.), *European Perspectives on Psychology*, Vol. 2. Sussex: Wiley.

Gjerde, P. F. (1983). Attentional capacity dysfunction and arousal in schizophrenia. *Psychological Bulletin*, 93(1), 57–72.

Glass, D. C., & Singer, J. E. (1972). Behavioral aftereffects of unpredictable and uncontrollable aversive events. *American Scientist,* 60, 457–465.

Goldstein, G., & Zubin, J. (1990). Neuropsychological differences between young and old schizophrenics with and without associated neurological dysfunction. *Schizophrenia Research,* 3, 117–126.

Green, M., & Walker, E. (1984). Susceptibility to backward masking in schizophrenic patients with positive or negative symptoms. *American Journal of Psychiatry,* 141(10), 1273–1275.

Green, M., & Walker, E. (1985). Neuropsychological performance and positive and negative symptoms in schizophrenia. *Journal of Abnormal Psychology,* 94(4) 460–469.

Halstead, W. C. (1947). *Brain and intelligence; a quantitative study of the frontal lobes.* Chicago: University of Chicago Press.

Hasher, L., & Zacks, R. T. (1979). Automatic and effortful processes in memory. *Journal of Experimental Psychology: General,* 108, 356–388.

Kay, S. R., Opler, L. A., & Fiszbein, A. (1986). Significance of positive and negative syndromes in chronic schizophrenia. *British Journal of Psychiatry,* 149, 439–448.

Klonoff, H., Fibiger, C. H., & Hutton, G. H. (1970). Neuropsychological patterns in chronic schizophrenia. *Journal of Nervous and Mental Disease,* 150(4), 291–300.

Koh, S. D., Kayton, L., & Peterson, R. A. (1976). Affective encoding and consequent remembering in schizophrenic young adults. *Journal of Abnormal Psychology,* 85, 156–166.

Kolakowska, T., Jambor, W. K., & Ardern, M. (1985). Schizophrenia with good and poor outcome: III. Neurological "soft" signs, cognitive impairment and their clinical significance. *British Journal of Psychiatry,* 146, 348–357.

Korchin, S. (1964). Anxiety and cognition. In E. Scheerer (Ed.), *Cognition: Theory, research, promise.* New York: Harper & Row.

Liddle, P. F. (1987a) The symptoms of chronic schizophrenia: a re-examination of the positive-negative dichotomy. *British Journal of Psychiatry,* 151, 145–151.

Liddle, P. F. (1987b) Schizophrenic syndromes, cognitive performance and neurological dysfunction. *Psychological Medicine,* 16, 49–57.

Liddle, P. F., & Barnes, T. R. E. (1990). Syndromes of chronic schizophrenia. *British Journal of Psychiatry,* 157, 558–561.

Liddle, P. F., & Morris, D. L. (1991). Schizophrenic syndromes and frontal lobe performance. *British Journal of Psychiatry,* 158, 340–345.

Luteijn, F., & van der Ploeg, F. A. E. (1983). Gröninger Intelligentie Test. Lisse, The Netherlands: Swets & Zeitlinger.

Meichenbaum, D., & Cameron, R. (1973). Training schizophrenics to talk to themselves: A means of developing attentional controls. *Behavior Therapy,* 4, 515–534.

Meiselman, K. C. (1970). Broadening dual modality cue utilization in chronic nonparanoid schizophrenics. *Journal of Consulting and Clinical Psychology,* 41, 447–453.

Miller, J. G. (1960). Information overload and psychopathology. *American Journal of Psychiatry,* 116, 695–704.

Nelson, H. E. (1976). A modified card sorting test sensitive to frontal lobe deficits. *Cortex,* 12, 313–324.

Nuechterlein, K. H., & Dawson, M. E. (1984a). Information processing and attentional functioning in the developmental course of schizophrenic disorders. *Schizophrenia Bulletin,* 10(2), 160–203.

Nuechterlein, K. H., & Dawson, M. E. (1984b). A heuristic vulnerability-stress model of schizophrenic episodes. *Schizophrenia Bulletin,* 10(2), 300–312.

Olbrich, R., & Mussgay, L. (1990). Reduction of schizophrenic deficits by cognitive training: an evaluative study. *European Archives of Psychiatry and Neurological Sciences,* 239, 366–369.

Pribram, K. H., & McGuinness, D. (1975). Arousal, activation, and effort in the control of attention. *Psychological Review,* 82(2), 116–149.

Rey, A. (1964). *L'examen clinique en psychologie.* Paris: Presses Universitaires de France.

Rosvold, H. E., Mirsky, A., Sarason, I., Bransbome, E. D., Jr., & Beck, L. H. (1956). A continuous performance test of brain damage. *Journal of Consulting Psychology,* 20, 343–350.

Sanders, A. F. (1983). Towards a model of stress and human performance. *Acta Psychologica,* 53, 61–97.

Schmand, B. A. (1991). The energetics of cognition in psychosis. Doctoral dissertation, Rijksuniversiteit Utrecht, Utrecht.

Schwartz, S. (1975). Individual differences in cognition: Some relationships between personality and memory. *Journal of Research in Personality,* 9, 217–225.

Shiffrin, R. M., & Schneider, W. (1977). Controlled and automatic human information processing: II. Perceptual learning, automatic attending and a general theory. *Psychological Review,* 84, 127–189.

Silverman, J, (1972). Stimulus intensity modulation and psychological disease. *Psychopharmacologica,* 24, 42–80.

Smith, A. (1964). Mental deterioration in chronic schizophrenia. *Journal of Nervous and Mental Disease,* 139, 479–487.

Stroop, J. R. (1935). Studies of interference in serial verbal reactions. *Journal of Experimental Psychology,* 12, 242–248.

Tucker, D. M., & Williamson, P. A. (1984). Asymmetric neural control systems in human self-regulation. *Psychological Review,* 81(2), 185–215.

Waddington, J. L., Youssef, H. A., & Kinsella, A. (1990). Cognitive dysfunction in schizophrenia followed up over 5 years, and its longitudinal relationship to the emergence of tardive dyskinesia. *Psychological Medicine,* 20, 835–842.

Wagner, B. R. (1968). The training of attending and abstracting responses in chronic schizophrenics. *Journal of Experimental Research in Personality,* 3, 77–88.

Wagman, A. M. I., Heinrichs, D. W., & Carpenter, W. T., Jr. (1987). Deficit and non-deficit forms of schizophrenia: Neuropsychological evaluation. *Psychiatry Research, 22*, 319–330.

Walley, R. E., & Weiden, T. D. (1973). Lateral inhibition and cognitive masking. *Psychological Review,* 80, 284–302.

Wechsler, D. (1958). The measurement and appraisal of adult intelligence. (4th ed.). Baltimore: Williams & Wilkins.

• 9 •

Cognitive-Behavioral Treatments for Schizophrenia: Evolving Rehabilitation Techniques

Robert K. Heinssen and Brian J. Victor

It has been more than 20 years since cognitive scientists first shook B.F. Skinner's black box. The "cognitive revolution" (Mahoney & Arnkoff, 1978) has radically changed the way behavior therapists conceptualize human thought and action. The mechanistic conditioning model of the late 1950s, with its emphasis on environmental determinism, no longer dominates. In its place stands a contemporary learning paradigm that portrays human beings as dynamic information-seeking and -processing organisms.

The shift to a cognitive framework has transformed many behavioral treatments, including rehabilitation strategies for schizophrenia. Although psychosocial treatments for this disorder have retained elements from earlier behavioral systems (i.e., operant conditioning and social learning approaches), many contemporary behavioral treatment approaches reflect an information-processing perspective (e.g., Bellack, Turner et al., 1984; Brenner, 1989; Hogarty et al., 1986; Wallace & Liberman, 1985). This new conceptual model emphasizes the interdependence of cognitive operations and motor skills in adaptive functioning (Liberman, Mueser et al., 1986; Wallace, 1982, 1984). Since a variety of factors potentially contribute to schizophrenic patients' poor motor skills, the goal of treatment is to identify relevant cognitive/motor deficiencies and then introduce strategies to surmount them.

This work was supported in part by a Young Investigator Award to Dr. Heinssen from the National Alliance for Research on Schizophrenia and Depression. The authors thank Lawrence Conroy, Lenore Fagen, Brenda Schneider, Dr. Bert Nayfack, Dr. Dexter M. Bullard, Jr., and the staff of the Chestnut Lodge Research Institute for their support in the writing of this chapter.

While the cognitive perspective has helped generate a new rehabilitation model for schizophrenia, it is not yet clear how information-processing concepts are best operationalized in skills training programs. At least two strategies warrant consideration. The first approach would adapt for clinical use certain tests designed to study cognitive operations in the laboratory (Spaulding et al., 1986). Experimental tasks would be used to assess a client's baseline processing capacity and later to train skills such as attention, concentration, discrimination, and problem solving. The appeal lies in this method's relationship to existing procedures for studying information processing and its similarity to training techniques developed for brain-injured patients (Gummow, Miller, & Duftman, 1983). However, the validity of this approach has been questioned. In Chapter 3 of this volume, for example, Erikson argues that the cognitive operations studied in experimental situations may bear little resemblance to information processing in natural settings. Thus, experimental training tasks may not exercise the particular cognitive skills required to function effectively in social and occupational environments. If this is the case, laboratory-based procedures (as they are currently conceived) will have minimal relevance to existing skills training programs.

The second method for operationalizing cognitive constructs is closely tied to traditional behavioral assessment and treatment procedures. This strategy expands the scope of behavior analysis to include cognitive operations embedded in specific daily activities. Clinicians first catalog the cognitive mechanisms involved in particular adaptive behaviors, evaluate patients on these dimensions, and then treat observed processing deficits like other behavioral targets. Cognitive disabilities are ameliorated through conventional skills training procedures, thereby ensuring consistency of treatment methods across cognitive and behavioral domains. One example of this approach is provided by Wallace and his colleagues (Wallace, 1982; Wallace & Liberman, 1985), who have described a similar process for identifying and treating social-processing deficits in schizophrenic patients.

The major attraction of this pragmatic approach is that cognitive phenomena are evaluated in a more natural context. This improves the likelihood that relevant processing mechanisms will be surveyed and that training procedures can be directed precisely at situation-specific deficits. However, this model has not been rigorously tested, and there are no guidelines for evaluating information-processing phenomena as they occur in everyday behaviors. Furthermore, it is unclear how certain cognitive operations (e.g., attention, short-term memory, concept formation) can be trained within a traditional skills development model. Many important aspects of this method are unexplored and deserve further investigation.

This chapter describes efforts to introduce cognitive principles into an existing behavioral treatment system. The Sullivan House Rehabilitation Program at Chestnut Lodge Hospital (Rockville, Maryland) prepares schizophrenic inpatients for full reintegration into the community by emphasizing the acquisition of adaptive instrumental skills. Although a token economy structures the milieu (see Paul & Lentz, 1977), many treatment procedures have been modified according to contemporary cognitive theories of schizophrenia. One component of the Sullivan House program, the vocational training module, best illustrates the translation of cognitive principles into effective behavioral treatments.

Cognition and Behavior in Vocational Retraining

The vocational training program at Sullivan House evolved to address the needs of a specific group of individuals; chronically ill schizophrenic patients who have been hospitalized for many years. Generally, residents lack prior occupational experience, and vocational aspirations, if present at all, are frequently unrealistic (e.g., "I want to be a movie star"). Motivation for employment is usually low, and difficulties such as high distractibility, limited concentration and memory, ineffective decision making, and poor social skills make many patients unsuitable for conventional retraining programs. Consequently, a vocational module was developed that seeks to "jump-start" interest and motivation for occupational endeavors, while at the same time addressing a broad array of cognitive, motoric, and interpersonal deficits.

DEFINING THE WORK PROJECT

Several assumptions influenced the development of a meaningful work program for our patients. These included:

1. The vocational project should create a marketable product.
2. The project should promote interaction with the outside community.
3. All work tasks should be reducible to concrete procedures.

4. Job responsibilities should be consistent, predictable, and require daily attendance.
5. The training program should teach marketable skills.
6. Employee-trainees should receive compensation for work effort.

The program needed a niche within the local economy where patients could furnish services that were otherwise unavailable. Such a role would promote a sense of accomplishment in patient-employees, and transactions with outside consumers would reestablish a positive connection with the community. An organic vegetable garden proved an effective solution, since a survey of area businesses revealed a surplus of health food stores but a shortage of organically grown produce. Several additional features made the organic garden an attractive work project: (a) interest among patients and vendors alike, (b) numerous concrete, repetitive duties requiring daily attention, (c) a low-technology quality that needs no sophisticated equipment, (d) the opportunity for patients to learn a unique craft, and (e) the availability of arable land at Chestnut Lodge for summer planting and a greenhouse for winter crops.

A small entrepreneurial venture was launched in June 1990, and the project has continued uninterrupted. To date, 31 patients have participated in the Sullivan House Organic Gardening Project, selling several tons of organically grown produce to local markets. Gardening sessions have been offered approximately 10 times each week throughout this period, providing many opportunities for patients to participate in the training program. Meetings have been structured to last no longer than 45 minutes, and the patient/staff ratio is kept low (i.e., 3:1) to guarantee adequate attention from clinicians. Work sessions are complemented by a mandatory weekly discussion group. Here patient-employees receive verbal recognition for their efforts and explore a variety of issues concerning the gardening program (e.g., what to plant, when to harvest, relevant job assignments, and so forth). Work accomplishments are further recognized during weekly unit meetings, where patients are praised copiously by Sullivan House staff members (psychiatrists, psychologists, social workers, and nursing personnel) for their vocational exertions.

Because the organic garden generates a small amount of revenue, each patient-employee can be compensated in two different currencies. "Sullivan Dollars," which are negotiable in the unit's token economy, are distributed after each training session, and U.S. dollars are distributed bimonthly in the form of a paycheck. Not surprisingly, financial compensation has proven to be a powerful incentive for many patients, and the availability of income often inspires better work performance. In fact, patients are frequently motivated to advance from the entry level position (apprentice) to higher placements (worker or manager) after discovering that the more responsible positions pay at a higher rate.

Cognitive Assessment Procedures

McGlashan, Heinssen, and Fenton (1989) have discussed the importance of "friendly" learning environments in treatment programs for schizophrenic patients. Such a milieu places minimal demands on a patient's information processing and supports residual cognitive resources during training sessions. The initial step in creating this condition is to analyze carefully the cognitive and behavioral operations involved in the training process. Thus, the first task in developing the gardening project was to define the information processing skills involved in gardening activities.

Task Analysis. The Behavior Analytic Technique (Goldfried & D'Zurilla, 1969) was used to identify the cognitive and motoric skills required to perform various gardening tasks. For example, the sequential operations involved in the watering of a greenhouse tomato plant were articulated by watching an experienced gardener perform the action repeatedly. Although it was relatively easy to classify constituent motor responses, it was necessary to question the expert closely concerning covert procedures (e.g., "How did you decide to perform that particular action just then?"). Careful examination of the watering process revealed that the activity consists of cognitive components (viz., attention, perceptual discrimination, concept sorting, short-term memory, and decision making) and motoric skills (viz., handling tools and pouring water precisely) that are coordinated when performing the task. Similar behavioral assessments enumerated the cognitive and motoric elements of seed planting, leaf spraying, weeding, and pruning.

Functional Assessment. Although task analysis specified the skills necessary to perform gardening tasks competently, this procedure disclosed nothing about patients' proficiency in performing these assignments. Consequently, several clients participated in functional assessment sessions (Cohen & Anthony, 1984) with the intent of cataloging deficits that can interfere with gardening performance. Information-processing skills and motor behaviors were evaluated in the work setting, and salient environmental features (i.e, those that either enhanced or diminished performance) were defined.

Data from the watering test revealed common cognitive difficulties. Many individuals were unable to focus on the job at hand, and they were easily distracted by the actions of others in the work area. Furthermore, few patients were able to master visual (e.g., "Is the soil light or dark?") or tactile (e.g., "Is the soil moist or dry?") discrimination trials consistently. Memory lapses were common, with patients demonstrating a tendency to lose track of task demands. Decision making (i.e., whether to water the plant or not) was generally impulsive and erratic. Likewise, behavioral and social deficiencies were observed in manipulating tools (e.g., pouring water accurately, refilling containers) and in interacting appropriately with work partners. In general, patients were easily overwhelmed by the watering test, became discouraged quickly, and passively withdrew from the assessment situation. Similar responses were observed on the functional tests for seed planting, leaf spraying, weeding, and pruning.

Results from the various functional analyses detailed cognitive impairments that clearly hampered effective behavioral performance. Not surprisingly, processing seemed to deteriorate most rapidly in unstructured, "noisy" settings, where extraneous stimuli competed for the client's attention. We surmised that the bustle and hubbub of the work setting (an operational greenhouse) proved too great a distraction. Training exercises, in order to be effective, would have to take place under less demanding conditions. Environmental manipulations similar to those suggested by Liberman and his colleagues (Liberman, Nuechterlein & Wallace, 1982) were subsequently introduced into the workplace to reduce information-processing requirements. This intervention represented the first component of the cognitive remediation process.

Cognitive Remediation Techniques

ENVIRONMENTAL ASPECTS OF COGNITIVE REHABILITATION

The initial task in cognitive retraining is to create an atmosphere that facilitates the client's attention and concentration. Specifically, the training site should be free of distracting elements and rich in orienting, task-relevant stimuli. These principles were applied to the greenhouse by selecting a private, quiet location for training and by clearing the spot of all extraneous materials. In addition, to foster attentional capacity and reduce memory requirements, posters bearing pertinent information about gardening procedures were hung in the training area. These prosthetic instruments, placed prominently in the training location, contained essential information that was written in a clear and abbreviated fashion. These features (visual prominence, linguistic clarity, and brevity) allowed rehabilitation clinicians to reorient distracted patients easily during training sessions, and helped clients keep track of task demands during rotating cognitive exercises.

Four posters were eventually developed, each focusing on a different gardening procedure—planting, watering, spraying, and pruning. The "Expert Watering" poster illustrates how cognitive elements derived from the task analysis were introduced during training sessions. To become expert at watering, for example, patients are instructed to (a) gather specific perceptual data (e.g., "Look at the soil"), (b) perform discrimination trials (e.g., "Is it light or dark?"), (c) retain two pieces of information simultaneously (i.e., color, moisture level), and (d) decide on an appropriate behavioral response. Posters are used at the onset of training to introduce a cognitive perspective on work performance, and later to highlight the relationship of one molecular processing skill to another.

SHAPING MOLECULAR COGNITIVE SKILLS.

A response acquisition model (Bandura, 1969) was developed to establish and consolidate processing skills absent from a patient's cognitive repertoire. Cognitive operations are addressed sequentially, according to the hierarchies revealed in the task analyses. For the watering module, perceptual discrimination is addressed before short-term memory or decision-making operations. Skills training is done in an instructional format and includes the techniques of (a) instruction and coaching, (b) modeling correct responses, (c) rehearsal and corrective feedback, and (d) contingent reinforcement (Bellack & Hersen, 1979).

The actual training begins with an explanation: clinicians first discuss with patients the importance of attention, memory, and decision making in gardening operations, and later describe the treatment process. For example, the therapist might state, "Greenhouse gardening involves many details. A person must pay attention to little things like the color of soil or how moist a pot is. You have to remember these facts to make correct decisions, like whether a plant needs to be watered or should be left alone. Today we'll practice observation skills as the first step in expert watering." Verbal instructions then describe how a particular skill is performed: "You need to look at the pot carefully to determine the color of the soil. Focus your attention right here, by the roots, to see whether the dirt is light colored or dark."

Cognitive skills are operationalized to facilitate modeling and rehearsal procedures. For example, preparations for discrimination trials include filling 20 identical pots with soil. Half are watered heavily and half are dried thoroughly to create sets of dark/wet and light/dry containers. These vessels are intermingled prior to the training exercise. Clinicians demonstrate (i.e., model) visual discrimination skills by sorting pots into "light" and "dark" categories, verbalizing the process in the following manner:

> "Ok, now I am going to separate these pots into two groups: pots that have light-colored soil and pots that have dark soil. I will place light-colored pots here by the sign that says 'Light.' Dark pots go here by the sign that says 'Dark.' Let's look at the first container. You see, this soil is pale, almost the color of clay. Since it's a light color I put it by the 'Light' sign. Let's inspect another. Ok, now this one is different. See how black this dirt is? This one goes in the 'Dark' pile. I'll just keep sorting them, noticing the differences in color each time."

The modeling process continues until all 20 vessels are correctly categorized. Once this is accomplished, the clinician invites active participation through skill rehearsal and feedback. Clients are encouraged to verbalize their actions while sorting the pots. The clinician provides feedback by highlighting accurate choices (e.g., "Very good. That's exactly right; the soil is black, so this one goes with the other 'Dark' pots"). Negative comments are avoided, since these are particularly disruptive to schizophrenic patients (Garmezy, 1952). The rehearsal and feedback phase continues until the patient displays reliable visual discrimination (90 percent accuracy, or 36 correct responses) on two consecutive sorting trials.

The training process resumes after visual sorting is mastered, this time emphasizing tactile discrimination. Instructional techniques are identical to those just described: the clinician first uses the "Expert Watering" poster to introduce the new operation and explain its significance. Modeling follows, as the clinician inserts a finger into the pot to check moisture level and then sorts vessels into "Moist" and "Dry" categories. The modeling is immediately followed by a rehearsal and feedback phase, which continues until mastery (90 percent accuracy) is demonstrated on two successive trials.

Decision-making skills are honed last of all. Although procedures during this phase are comparable to those described above, some changes are necessary due to unique task characteristics. For example, while visual and tactile sorting procedures can be operationalized, decision making is a more abstract process, involving memory and reasoning functions. These capacities are not easily reduced to constituent behaviors, and they cannot be represented by physical objects. Consequently, instructional posters are used to illustrate decision-making algorithms and to enhance memory and executive functions. Clinicians refer frequently to the "Expert Watering" poster when modeling decision-making skills: "Ok, let's check the poster. Is the soil light or dark? It looks light. Is it wet or dry? It feels dry. Now put the facts together and make a decision. It's light and dry so the correct decision is to water the plant." Patients are encouraged to mimic overt verbalization during the early phase of training but to gradually fade verbal self-instructions over time (Meichenbaum & Cameron, 1973). Practice in decision making ceases when accuracy (90 percent correct response rate) is achieved on two consecutive trials.

Decision-making skills are harder to master than discrimination abilities. Numerous practice sessions, spaced over several days, are necessary before patients render judgments reliably. Ultimately, however, these skills can be learned and the majority of patients graduate to the next component of training, the acquisition of molar work behaviors.

SHAPING MOLAR BEHAVIORS

The response acquisition model was also applied to motor skills, establishing continuity of treatment across cognitive and motor behaviors. Training sessions were moved to the general work area for this phase, permitting patients to practice cognitive operations in a less-protected environment and to acquire motor skills in the target work setting. For example, clinicians introduce the motor aspects of expert watering by first reviewing the importance of inspection and judgment skills and then describing watering methods: "Don't disturb the roots of the plant when you're watering. They can be injured if water is poured directly on them, so aim the stream here, by the wall of the pot." The clinician then models the watering technique repeatedly (where to pour, how quickly, and how much water to disburse), using the greenhouse tomato plants to demonstrate.

Although the clients' primary task is to observe during the modeling period, patients are also asked to assume an active role in the process. The patient is required to make judgments about the need for watering and to guide the clinician's actions accordingly (e.g., "This one is dark and moist so you should leave it alone"). This accomplishes two objectives. First, patients practice inspection and judgment abilities in a more stressful environment (the actual greenhouse), thereby "cultivating" cognitive efficiency in a more stimulating situation. Second, generalization of learned skills is promoted by requiring patients to perform cognitive operations outside of the initial training site. Similar strategies have been suggested to increase the generalizability of acquired motor behaviors (Bellack & Morrison, 1985), and these techniques may have relevance to cognitive skills as well.

The rehearsal-feedback stage for the watering technique is initiated once a client's cognitive skills appear accurate and reliable. Patients are asked not only to verbalize the decision-making process, but also to perform requisite motor behaviors themselves. Verbal prompts are gradually faded as judgments become more exact, and the clinician recedes further into the background as behavioral responses became more effective. An individual's "apprenticeship" concludes when 20 consecutive plants are watered correctly (i.e., 20 appropriate judgments with proper technique on each occasion). The client graduates to "worker" status at this point, and supervision and reinforcement schedules changed from continuous to intermittent.

Modifying Expectations and Beliefs

Initial results from the gardening project were indeed promising: patients appeared interested in training tasks, they participated regularly in practice sessions, and most acquired new skills at a slow but steady pace. Unfortunately, performance was yoked to staff monitoring, and patients' response rates dropped precipitously whenever supervision ceased. Faulty learning did not appear to be the central problem, since the new skills could be performed upon demand. Other factors were sought to account for the observed deficits in initiative and perseverance and to explain why learned behaviors were suppressed in the workplace. Clinical data obtained outside of the work situation suggested the influence of other cognitive variables upon the patients, namely exaggerated expectations of failure and fixed beliefs about personal ineffectiveness.

Expectations of Failure. Sadly, many patients who enter the rehabilitation program have an extensive history of instrumental failure. Premorbid functioning is generally poor across social, scholastic, and occupational spheres and subsequent deterioration has compounded patients' feelings of demoralization. Data disclosed to social workers and psychotherapists established that most patients anticipated an inability to apply new skills and expected a variety of negative consequences for poor performance (e.g., embarrassment, ridicule, and shame). These anticipatory fears immobilize patients whenever external support is lacking, and this explains the poor initiative and perseverance observed on unsupervised work activities. Consequently, new elements were introduced into the training program to counteract expectations of failure and to foster a healthier perception of personal effectiveness.

Rehabilitation procedures were revised to emphasize positive learning experiences and to generate healthier estimates of self-efficacy. Two strategies were employed to achieve this goal. First, training protocols were manipulated to maximize the likelihood of correct responses. Second, clinicians began actively attributing successful results to patients' efforts and skills. These modifications were introduced throughout the rehabilitation program, starting with treatment planning.

Data from neuropsychological assessments is used to improve the structure of initial training sessions (Erikson & Binder, 1986). Attention, concentration, and reasoning skills are evaluated to determine optimum conditions regarding the duration of meetings, the frequency of appointments, and the complexity of learning tasks. Occasionally, it is necessary to assign distractible patients to 10-minute training sessions that present simplified tasks (e.g., "Which of these two pots looks darker to you?"). Concrete reinforcers are delivered immediately to these individuals to sustain interest and motivation for training exercises (e.g., "Very good. Take a sip of your soda before we try it again"). In most cases, however, such intense conditioning of attention is not necessary.

By accommodating to each patient's skill/deficit profile, this approach amplifies mastery experiences early on and thereby introduces positive expectations regarding learning potential. "Success momentum" is preserved by linking increases in task difficulty (longer training sessions and higher processing demands) to improvements in patients' behavioral competence. Although this tends to prolong the training process, most patients show increased self-confidence as a result.

Clinicians nurture feelings of personal effectiveness throughout this process by enhancing the corrective feedback offered to patients. For example, clinicians respond to accurate responses with statements that emphasize the patient's growing competence: "You've mastered this nicely; it's a challenge, but you're picking up the skills." Conversely, incorrect responses are reframed with coping statements: "Well, that one wasn't right, but no problem. Anyone can make a mistake when learning something new." Although these subtle prompts are sufficient to change expectancy sets in many individuals, they are not universally effective. More direct methods proved necessary to foster feelings of empowerment in some patients.

Fixed Dysfunctional Beliefs. Each patient is routinely interviewed by Sullivan House treatment personnel to evaluate the overall effectiveness of the rehabilitation program. These discussions have revealed a common feature among patients who do not respond to the initial cognitive reframing exercise. Rigid, self-limiting beliefs are often articulated by these individuals and are adamantly maintained even in the presence of contrary evidence. The strength and nature of these maladaptive convictions (e.g., "I'm telling you, I'm just no good at working. I've never been, and I never will be") suggest a link to the persistent behavioral deficits observed in the vocational setting. Consequently, methods from Beck's cognitive therapy (Beck, 1976; Beck et al., 1979; Beck & Weishaar, 1989) were incorporated to address these dysfunctional beliefs directly. The intention was to improve patients' poor initiative and perseverance by first modifying relevant thoughts and attitudes through cognitive restructuring.

Described in very basic terms, cognitive therapy is an approach to treatment that emphasizes the influence of thoughts, beliefs, and self-statements on a person's affect and behavior (Bedrosian & Beck, 1980). According to this paradigm, actions are determined by personal convictions, and the difference between behavioral effectiveness and incompetence lies primarily in an individual's expectations and beliefs. Certain opinions (e.g., "Things always work out for the best") may encourage a confident, extraverted style, while others (e.g., "The world is a dangerous place") foster anxious and avoidant responses. Not surprisingly, the primary goal of cognitive therapy is to help a patient become aware of self-limiting assumptions and then supplant these with new and more functional meaning structures (Perris, 1989).

The cognitive approach is a highly verbal, interactive treatment that requires patients to reflect upon their actions, monitor their thought process, and evaluate rationally the reasonableness of their personal interpretations. As such, cognitive therapy is a cognitively demanding procedure that assumes the integrity of basic information-processing mechanisms. At first this approach may seem unsuited for schizophrenia, where deficits of attention, concentration, memory, and abstract reasoning are common. However, cognitive therapy techniques can be utilized with schizophrenic patients with certain provisions (Bowers, 1989; Hibbard et al., 1987; Perris, 1989). These include (a) evaluating maladaptive cognitions in the context of specific behavioral tasks, (b) simplifying dysfunctional thoughts and beliefs to the patient's level of understanding, and (c) maintaining a behavioral focus during the early stage of treatment. It is possible to "concretize" Beck's standard approach by applying these principles in a manner that addresses the processing deficits of our patients. The following case illustrates this strategy.

> Rita, a 22-year-old schizophrenic woman, was enrolled in the Organic Gardening Project. Although she performed many tasks effectively, Rita was unable to initiate or sustain work performance without supervision. Several interviews with her social worker (Mrs. B) enabled Rita to explore her difficulties in the vocational program, including her feelings of demoralization and helplessness regarding her occupational potential. Rita recounted past failures with vocational training and summarized these experiences as follows: "I guess I'm just too dumb to learn anything new. I'll never be good enough to get a real job."
>
> Mrs. B emphasized the personal nature of Rita's account and presented other important facts for discussion. For example, rehabilitation clinicians reported that Rita was not only capable of learning new skills, but that her overall progress suggested an eventual promotion to the hospital's general work program. Rita's negative thoughts, however, seemed to lower her self-confidence and limit her effectiveness when she worked alone. Mrs. B suggested that Rita might feel more comfortable in the greenhouse if she "tried on some new thoughts" while working. Specifically, Rita was instructed to remind herself of her positive qualities several times during each work session.
>
> Rita agreed to try this experiment and she and Mrs. B crafted a brief,

> but highly relevant, statement to counteract her negative interpretations. Mrs. B operationalized the cognitive restructuring procedure by (a) reproducing the adaptive self-statement ("I am a good worker") on several index cards, (b) posting these in Rita's bedroom and in the greenhouse, and (c) defining a daily schedule for "thought practice." Rita agreed to repeat the message aloud once in the morning after making her bed and once prior to retiring. In addition, rehabilitation clinicians prompted Rita to rehearse the self-statement before, during, and immediately following vocational training sessions. Other aspects of Rita's vocational program remained unchanged.
>
> Rehabilitation clinicians reported improvement in sustained performance following several sessions of this form of in vivo cognitive restructuring. Self-initiated behaviors were slower to develop, but they did appear after several weeks of consistent "thought practice." Rita was eventually promoted to a managerial position within the Gardening Project and she later moved on to other jobs in the hospital work program. At discharge several months later, Rita spontaneously reported confidence in obtaining outside employment because "After all, I'm a very good worker."

This case illustrates how cognitive psychotherapy techniques may be adapted for use with schizophrenic patients by carefully attending to information-processing limitations and specific task demands. Working collaboratively, patient and therapist can condense self-limiting beliefs to a brief but cogent phrase. An equally terse counterstatement is generated and introduced into the rehabilitation process as concretely as possible. The adaptive thought is then treated like other behavioral targets and is repeatedly practiced along with other necessary skills. Clinical experience so far suggests that this combined cognitive-behavioral approach—cognitive remediation, cognitive restructuring, and motor skills training—can successfully reverse self-defeating attributions and foster durable vocational skills in some chronic schizophrenic patients.

Effectiveness of the Cognitive-Behavioral Model: Preliminary Data

The Organic Gardening Project was originally conceived as a pump-priming venture, an intervention designed to foster patients' interest in further vocational training. It was hoped that patients enrolled in this project would eventually move on to the hospital's general work program to develop additional job skills and to acquire further occupational experience. Success with the Gardening Project was monitored and this information was used to evaluate the effectiveness of more advanced vocational rehabilitation.

For the purpose of comparison, a control sample matched the first 10 participants in the gardening program with other Chestnut Lodge patients for diagnosis, gender, and age. The two samples were later evaluated on several measures of vocational adjustment. All patients received comprehensive treatment during the study period (May 1 to December 31, 1990), including pharmacotherapy, individual psychotherapy, and supportive family counseling. Individuals in the control condition received traditional milieu therapy instead of participating in the gardening project.

The gardening sample was composed entirely of patients within the schizophrenia spectrum: 30 percent paranoid type, 60 percent undifferentiated type, and 10 percent schizoaffective disorder. Men ($n = 7$) dominated this relatively young cohort ($M = 31.6$ years). The control sample was similarly constituted regarding diagnosis (50 percent paranoid type, 40 percent undifferentiated type, 10 percent schizoaffective disorder), gender (70 percent men), and age ($M = 29.9$ years). A review of medication records indicated that the two samples received equivalent doses of neuroleptic and mood-stabilizing compounds during the period of interest.

An analysis of archival data revealed additional similarities between the two groups. As summarized in table 9.1, patients frequently displayed the first signs of illness in their midteens and required psychiatric hospitalization shortly thereafter. By the time of this study, all patients had been ill for over a decade, experiencing many prior hospitalizations. Thus, both samples could be considered chronic and treatment-refractory. However, results from standardized tests of intellectual functioning indicated fewer cognitive resources among individuals in the gardening sample, suggesting a greater degree of overall impairment among these patients.

Premorbid work accomplishments were evaluated by applying the Acquisition of Skills and Interests Measure (Fenton & McGlashan, 1987; Harty et al. 1981). This instrument was used to assess an individual's highest level of occupational achievement and avocational activity prior to this study. Scores on this measure range from 0 (no occupational accomplishments/no curiosities or hobbies) to 4 (working at an occupation/active avocational interests). Patients in both groups demonstrated significant impairment on this di-

Table 9.1. Group Means and Significance Tests on Selected Illness Dimensions: Gardening Project Subjects and Matched Control Groups

Illness Dimension	*Treatment Condition*		$t(18)$	p
	Gardening Project (n = 10)	*Matched Control* (n = 10)		
Age at illness onset (years)	16.3	16.5	0.11	NS
Length of illness (years)	15.3	13.7	0.59	NS
Prior hospitalizations	10.3	7.2	1.62	NS
Full-scale IQ (index admission)	84.6	102.9	2.53	<.025
Premorbid work skills[a]	1.6	1.7	0.23	NS

a. Scores on promorbid work skills measure ranged from 0 (no skills) to 4 (normal skill levels).

mension (see table 9.1), with little evidence of previous occupational achievement. Work experience, if present at all, was usually limited to low-level jobs (e.g., fry cook, grocery clerk), and avocational pursuits were rare. This indifference toward occupational endeavors continued into the index hospitalization. At baseline assessment very few patients in the gardening (n = 2) or control (n = 3) conditions were involved in the hospital work program.

Patients enrolled in the Organic Gardening Project participated in approximately four training sessions per week for 29 weeks. Rehabilitation clinicians noticed a gradual improvement over time in job interest and work activity among treated subjects. Patients responded well to the training program, and appeared to enjoy the verbal and concrete rewards that were disbursed during training sessions, weekly discussion groups, and forays into the community. Furthermore, an important behavioral change was noted. While the proportion of patients enrolled in hospital jobs was similar at baseline, significant differences were observed between the two groups six months later (chi square [3, N = 20] = 10.56, $p < .01$). Eighty percent of the patients in the gardening group, for example, had obtained jobs in the hospital work program, while only 20 percent of the patients in the matched control sample held comparable positions. This represented a fourfold increase in work activity among patients in the gardening group and a concurrent decline in vocational training among control subjects.

The fact that considerable improvement was noted following only six months of vocational training indicates that the gardening project was effective in stimulating work interest and motivation. Furthermore, durable gains appear possible. A one-year followup assessment found the eight garden project alumni pursuing vocational goals either in the hospital work program ($n = 4$) or through community placements ($n = 4$).

While these results are encouraging, they do not necessarily confirm the efficacy of cognitive remediation procedures. The patients were exposed to numerous interventions that included several nonspecific strategies. Among these ambient features were (a) the novelty of a pilot treatment program, (b) enthusiastic and dedicated clinicians, (c) effective role models in the hospital and in the community, (d) placement in a genuine work setting, and (e) compensation for practicing new job skills. Each of these factors undoubtedly contributed to the overall treatment effect.

The gardening project also contained many unique elements that reflect the influence of a cognitive framework. With regard to information processing, a learning environment was created that focused and supported each patient's residual cognitive resources, while at the same time training increased processing efficiency. Furthermore, training exercises were titrated in order to minimize cognitive failures and foster sustained success. The project also sought to nurture new beliefs and expectations regarding work activities and to help patients generally develop more effective vocational schemata. Because these interventions were presented as a single treatment package, it is unclear which treatment elements contributed uniquely to overall outcome. Controlled "dismantling" studies (Kazdin, 1980; 1986) are required to determine the relative importance of the various ingredients (i.e., environmental prosthetics, processing exercises, and cognitive restructuring techniques) on vocational performance. Nonetheless, the findings suggest that such research is justified, since some aspect of our treatment package stimulated improvement in this sample of chronic schizophrenic patients.

Summary and Conclusions

The cognitive processing model provides a new way of understanding the rehabilitation process with schizophrenic patients. The major appeal of this paradigm is its conceptual elegance and the broad perspective it brings to assessment and treatment issues. However, it is not yet clear how the cognitive model is best operationalized for clinical practice. Many questions, both theoretical and practical, must be resolved before a reliable set of procedures can be added to the rehabilitation armamentarium. Controlled empirical research is clearly needed. Open clinical trials, however, can also contribute by exploring cognitive principles as they apply to existing treatment methods.

The program described in this chapter represents one attempt to introduce cognitive constructs into a behavioral rehabilitation framework. Cognitive assessment and treatment techniques were incorporated into a system that emphasizes operant and social learning principles, thereby bringing together three generations of behavioral treatment for schizophrenia. Experience illustrates that these strategies are not antithetical but can complement one another in a comprehensive approach to psychosocial treatment. Knowledge of processing deficits, for example, enabled us to plan interventions in a more sophisticated fashion. Conversely, the behavioral emphasis helped in translating cognitive operations into procedures amenable to skills training. The token economy provided an important backdrop for training efforts by effectively enhancing patients' motivation for rehabilitation activities. The combination of these three approaches resulted in an intervention that was effective for a sample of treatment-refractory patients, suggesting that this strategy warrants further study.

EXPANDING THE COGNITIVE REHABILITATION MODEL

Although initial efforts to "think cognitively" (Glass & Arnkoff, 1982) were based in the information processing framework, clinical data soon revealed the influence of other important covert factors. For example, cognitive problems such as erroneous beliefs (e.g., "I have no control over events") and diminished efficacy expectations (e.g., "Nothing I do will make a difference") fueled patients' demoralized feelings and contributed to hesitant and lethargic behavior during training sessions. It is not hard to imagine how such dysphoric ideas, if left untreated, could limit a patient's capacity to benefit from treatment. Furthermore, this type of cognitive dysfunction might affect how skills are applied outside of the training situation and might account for the meager generalization effects observed in many skills-training programs (Bellack & Morrison, 1985; Curran, Monti & Corriveau, 1985).

Cognitive therapy techniques could enhance rehabilitation efforts in at least two important ways. Deliberate attempts could be made early on to nurture a "learning mindset," with the goal of improving patients' receptivity to training procedures. This approach would require clinicians to assess dysfunctional attitudes about treatment and then help patients to replace these opinions with a facilitative outlook (e.g., "Everyone can learn new skills if they take their time"). Clinicians could also search for beliefs that might limit the generalization of skills (e.g., "This would never work in the real world") and then encourage patients to consider more adaptive hypotheses (e.g., "Maybe this will work and maybe it won't. I'll never know unless I try"). These activities would obviously expand the scope of rehabilitation endeavors, and clinicians would be required to model and shape cognitive-evaluative skills as well as behavioral responses.

A survey of the empirical literature illustrates that there is indeed growing interest in testing cognitive-behavioral methods with schizophrenic patients (Adams et al., 1981; Alford, 1986; Alford, Fleece & Rothblum, 1982; Beck, 1952; Bellack et al., 1984; Bentall, Higson & Lowe, 1987; Bowers, 1989; Brenner, 1989; Gumaer & Headspeth, 1985; Gummow, Miller & Duftman, 1983; Hansen, St. Lawrence & Christoff, 1985; Harty et al., 1981; Kingdon & Turkington, 1991; Lamontagne, Audet & Elie, 1983; Margolis & Shemberg, 1976; Meichenbaum & Cameron, 1973; Milton, Patwa & Hafner, 1978; Perris, 1989; Spaulding et al., 1986; Watts, Powell & Austin, 1973). Despite a tendency for small samples and variable experimental control, these studies suggest that cognitive treatment methods, including self-instructional training, cognitive restructuring, and problem solving, may be promising tools for psychiatric rehabilitation. Beneficial results were noted, for example, on a variety of treatment targets, including information-processing dimensions (e.g., attentional problems, distractibility, and memory dysfunction), positive symptoms (e.g., delusions and hallucinations) and problems in daily living (e.g., grooming, hygiene, and social interaction). The results presented in this chapter suggest the potential of cognitive therapy procedures for negative symptoms as well, including amotivation, avolition, and anhedonia. More often than not, the gains reported elsewhere were durable and they frequently generalized beyond the training situation. These results are impressive given that many interventions were quite brief (fewer than 10 sessions). If more is better, which in itself is an empirical question, then the potential for cognitively focused treatment may be substantial.

In conclusion, the current cognitive-behavioral treatment paradigm should be expanded to address multiple levels of cognitive impairment, as well as deficient behavioral skills (Heinssen & Glass, 1990). This requires that assessment and intervention strategies be modified to account for the information-processing operations relevant to particular actions and also to address the interpretive style that mediates a patient's behavioral response. Establishing guidelines for these procedures awaits further empirical research, but such efforts, it is hoped, will culminate in multilevel treatments that promote efficient information processing, positive expectancy sets, and adaptive behavioral responses. In this way the next generation of rehabilitation programs may be better equipped to address the multiple impairments that characterize the schizophrenic disorder.

References

Adams, H. E., Brantley, P. J., Malatesta, V., & Turkat, I. D. (1981). Modification of cognitive processes: A case study of schizophrenia. *Journal of Consulting and Clinical Psychology,* 49, 460–464.

Alford, B. A. (1986). Behavioral treatment of schizophrenic delusions: A single-case experimental analysis. *Behavior Therapy,* 17, 637–644.

Alford, G. S., Fleece, L., & Rothblum, E. (1982). Hallucinatory-delusional verbalizations: Modification in a chronic schizophrenic by self-control and cognitive restructuring. *Behavior Modification,* 6, 421–435.

American Psychiatric Association (1987). *Diagnostic and statistical manual of mental disorders* (3d Ed., Rev.). Washington, D.C.: APA.

Bandura, A. (1969). *Principles of behavior modification.* New York: Holt, Rinehart & Winston.

Beck, A. T. (1952). Successful outpatient psychotherapy of a chronic schizophrenic with a delusion based on borrowed guilt. *Psychiatry,* 15, 305–312.

Beck, A. T. (1976). *Cognitive therapy and the emotional disorders.* New York: International Universities Press.

Beck, A. T., Rush, A. J., Shaw, B. F., & Emery, G. (1979). *Cognitive therapy of depression.* New York: Guilford.

Beck, A. T., & Weishaar, M. (1989). Cognitive therapy. In A. Freeman, K. M. Simon, L. E. Beutler, & H. Arkowitz (Eds.), *Comprehensive handbook of cognitive therapy* (pp. 21–36). New York: Plenum.

Bedrosian, R. C., & Beck, A. T. (1980). Principles of cognitive therapy. In M. J. Mahoney (Ed.), *Psychotherapy process: current issues and future directions* (pp. 127–152). New York: Plenum.

Bellack, A. S., & Hersen, M. (Eds.). (1979). *Research and practice in social skills training.* New York: Plenum.

Bellack, A. S., & Morrison, R. L. (1985). Interpersonal dysfunction. In A. S. Bellack, M. Hersen & A. E. Kazdin (Eds.), *International handbook of behavior modification and therapy* (pp. 277–307). New York: Plenum.

Bellack, A. S., Turner, S. M., Hersen, M., & Luber, R. F. (1984). An examination of the efficacy of social skills training for chronic schizophrenic patients. *Hospital and Community Psychiatry,* 35, 1023–1028.

Bentall, R. P., Higson, P. J., & Lowe, C. F. (1987). Teaching self-instructions to chronic schizophrenic patients: Efficacy and generalization. *Behavioural Psychotherapy,* 15, 58–76.

Bowers, W. A. (1989). Cognitive therapy with inpatients. In A. Freeman, K. M. Simon, L. E. Beutler, & H. Arkowitz (Eds.), *Comprehensive handbook of cognitive therapy* (pp. 583–596). New York: Plenum.

Brenner, H. D. (1989). The treatment of basic psychological dysfunctions from a systemic point of view. *British Journal of Psychiatry,* 155, 74–83.

Cohen, B. F., & Anthony, W. A. (1984). Functional assessment in psychiatric rehabilitation. In A. S. Halpern & M. J. Fuhrer (Eds.), *Functional assessment in rehabilitation* (pp. 79–100). Baltimore: Paul Brooks.

Curran, J. P., Monti, P. M., & Corriveau, D. P. (1985). Treatment of schizophrenia. In A. S. Bellack, M. Hersen, & A. Kazdin (Eds.), *International handbook of behavior modification and therapy* (pp. 209–242). New York: Plenum.

Erikson, R. C., & Binder, L. M. (1986). Cognitive deficits among functionally psychotic patients: A rehabilitative perspective. *Journal of Clinical and Experimental Neuropsychology,* 8, 257–274.

Fenton, W. S., & McGlashan, T. H. (1987). Prognostic scale for chronic schizophrenia. *Schizophrenia Bulletin,* 13, 277–286.

Garmezy, N. (1952). Stimulus differentiation by schizophrenic and normal subjects under conditions of reward and punishment. *Journal of Personality,* 21, 353–376.

Glass, C. R., & Arnkoff, D. B. (1982). Think cognitively: Selected issues in cognitive assessment and therapy. In P. C. Kendall (Ed.), *Advances in cognitive-behavioral research and therapy* Vol. 1 (pp. 35–71). New York: Academic Press.

Goldfried, M. R., & D'Zurilla, T. J. (1969). A behavioral-analytic model for assessing competence. In C. D. Spielberger (Ed.), *Current topics in clinical and community psychology,* Vol. 1 (pp. 151–196). New York: Academic Press.

Gumaer, J., & Headspeth, T. (1985). Self-instructional training with an adolescent schizophrenic. *School Counselor,* 32, 371–380.

Gummow, L., Miller, P., & Duftman, R. (1983). Attention and brain injury: A case for cognitive rehabilitation of attentional deficits. *Clinical Psychology Review,* 3, 255–274.

Hansen, D. J., St. Lawrence, J. S., & Christoff, K. A. (1985). Effects of interpersonal problem-solving training with chronic aftercare patients on problem-solving component skills and effectiveness of solutions. *Journal of Consulting and Clinical Psychology,* 53, 167–174.

Harty, M., Cerney, M., Colson, P., Coyne, L., Frieswyk, S., Johnson, S. B., & Mortimer, R. (1981). Correlates of change and long term outcome: An exploratory study of intensively treated hospital patients. *Bulletin of the Menninger Clinic,* 45, 209–228.

Heinssen, R. K., & Glass, C. R. (1990). Social skills, social anxiety, and cognitive factors in schizophrenia. In H. Leitenberg (Ed.), Handbook of social and evaluation anxiety (pp. 325–355). New York: Plenum.

Hibbard, M. R., Gordon, W. A., Egelko, S., & Langer, K. (1987). Issues in the diagnosis and cognitive therapy of depression in brain-damaged individuals. In A. Freeman & V. Greenwood (Eds.), *Cognitive therapy: Applications in psychiatric and medical settings* (pp. 183–197). New York: Human Sciences Press.

Hogarty, G. E., Anderson, C. M., Reiss, D. J., Kornblith, S. J., Greenwald, D. P., Javna, C. D., & Madonia, M. J. (1986). Family psychoeducation, social skills training, and maintenance chemotherapy in the aftercare treatment of schizophrenia: I. One-year effects of a controlled study on relapse and expressed emotion. *Archives of General Psychiatry,* 43, 633–642.

Kazdin, A. E. (1980). *Research design in clinical psychology.* New York: Harper & Row.

Kazdin, A. E. (1986). Research designs and methodology. In S. L. Garfield & A. E. Bergin (Eds.), *Handbook of psychotherapy and behavior change* (3d Ed.; pp. 23–680). New York: John Wiley & Sons.

Kingdon, D. G., & Turkington, D. (1991). The use of cognitive behavior therapy with a normalizing rationale in schizophrenia: Preliminary report. *Journal of Nervous and Mental Disease,* 179, 207–211.

Lamontagne, Y., Audet, N., & Elie, R. (1983). Thought-stopping for delusions and hallucinations: A pilot study. *Behavioral Psychotherapy,* 11, 177–184.

Liberman, R. P., Mueser, K. T., Wallace, C. J., Jacobs, H. E., Eckman, T., & Massel, H. K. (1986). Training skills in the psychiatrically disabled: Learning coping and competence. *Schizophrenia Bulletin,* 12, 631–647.

Liberman, R. P., Nuechterlein, K. H., & Wallace, C. J. (1982). Social skills training and the nature of schizophrenia. In J. P. Curran & P. M. Monti (Eds.), *Social skills training: A practical handbook for assessment and treatment* (pp. 5–56). New York: Guilford.

McGlashan, T. H., Heinssen, R. K., & Fenton, W. S. (1989). Psychosocial treatment of negative symptoms in schizophrenia. In N. C. Andreasen (Ed.), *Modern problems in pharmacopsychiatry.* Vol. 24: *Schizophrenia: Positive and negative symptoms and syndromes* (pp. 175–200). Basel: Karger.

Mahoney, M. J., & Arnkoff, D. B. (1978). Cognitive and self-control therapies. In S. L. Garfield & A. E. Bergin (Eds.), *Handbook of psychotherapy and behavior change* (2d Ed., pp. 689–722). New York: John Wiley & Sons.

Margolis, R. B., & Shemberg, K. M. (1976). Cognitive self-instruction in process and reactive schizophrenics: A failure to replicate. *Behavior Therapy,* 7, 668–671.

Meichenbaum, D., & Cameron, R. (1973). Training schizophrenics to talk to themselves: A means of developing attentional controls. *Behavior Therapy,* 4, 515–534.

Milton, F., Patwa, V. K., & Hafner, R. J. (1978). Confrontation vs. belief modification in persistently deluded patients. *British Journal of Medical Psychology,* 51, 127–130.

Paul, G. L., & Lentz, R. J. (1977). *Psychosocial treatment of chronic mental patients.* Cambridge: Harvard University Press.

Perris, C. (1989). *Cognitive therapy with schizophrenic patients.* New York: Guilford.

Spaulding, W. D., Storms, L., Goodrich, V., & Sullivan, M. (1986). Applications of experimental psychopathology in psychiatric rehabilitation. *Schizophrenia Bulletin,* 12, 560–577.

Wallace, C. J. (1982). The social skills training project of the mental health clinical research center for the study of schizophrenia. In J. P. Curran & P. M. Monti (Eds.), *Social skills training: A practical handbook for assessment and treatment* (pp. 57–89). New York: Guilford.

Wallace, C. J. (1984). Community and interpersonal functioning in the course of schizophrenic disorders. *Schizophrenia Bulletin,* 10, 233–257.

Wallace, C. J., & Liberman, R. P. (1985). Social skills training for patients with schizophrenia: A controlled clinical trial. *Psychiatry Research,* 15, 239–247.

Watts, F. N., Powell, G. E., & Austin, S. V. (1973). The modification of abnormal beliefs. *British Journal of Medical Psychology,* 46, 359–363.

• 10 •
From Research to Practice: Considerations in Applying Cognitive Technology in the Public Mental Health System

Mark DeKraai and Peter G. Beeson

Cognitive assessment and treatment make up an exciting new technology that appears to have great potential benefit to persons with mental disorders and others with like conditions. The previous chapters have discussed the application of this new technology from occupational therapy and neuropsychological perspectives; examined its uses for assessment and treatment and rehabilitation programs; and explored its potential value for improving the lives of persons with schizophrenia, substance abuse problems, and other types of disorders. This new technology, however, is still considered experimental and its applications are to some extent confined to research settings. This chapter explores the issues related to the transfer of this technology from the research arena into the broader practice arena. First, we examine the general problem of knowledge dissemination and how it applies to cognitive assessment and treatment technology. Second, we explore the questions that must be answered before one can say with confidence that this technology is ready for dissemination. Third, we discuss some of the issues related to dissemination. And, finally, we present the results of a conference followup survey that provides some perspectives on the questions raised in previous sections.

This chapter is more food for thought than any definitive guidance about the transfer of this technology from the research arena to the practice arena. The chapter provides a framework for looking at issues and a series of questions that we hope will stimulate readers in their own analysis of the potential for cognitive assessment and treatment technology in improving the lives of persons with mental disorders.

From Knowledge Transfer to Knowledge Exchange

If the new knowledge generated by research is to make a positive difference in the lives of persons with mental disorders, this new knowledge must be incorporated into the skill repertoires of persons providing services. The traditional conception of such a research impact is depicted by a linear knowledge transfer model.

In this model, researchers identify the problem and design or conduct research to obtain knowledge about how the problem could be remedied; this knowledge is then transferred to those who apply the knowledge in addressing the problem. This model depicts a unidirectional flow of knowledge from an active knowledge producer to a passive knowledge consumer.

Experience has shown that the linear transfer model has a number of limitations. First, the issues addressed by researchers often are not the issues of concern to practitioners and policy makers. Second, there is a problem with the knowledge transfer component. Often research findings on public policy issues have been reported in basic science journals with little effort to communicate this knowledge directly to practitioners; and often information is couched in professional jargon that is inaccessible to the practitioner or policy maker. Third, there is the translatability problem: research results are often not in a form usable by the practitioner. A fourth problem with the linear transfer model is that researchers frequently fail to consider the feasibility of, or factors involved in, implementing the results.

The following illustration of the above-mentioned problems is provided by Davis (1979) in his widely cited A VICTORY (Ability, Values, Information, Circumstances, Timing, Obligation, Resistance, and Yield) model of sensitizing researchers to the practical aspects of knowledge utilization. In a midwestern state, a major study on institutional aftercare was conducted, and one of the findings was that when the same worker saw patients during hospitalization and after return to the community, the probability of readmission was significantly lowered. The researchers and consultants from the National Institute of Mental Health approached the commissioner responsible for county welfare departments and suggested a policy that would require county welfare workers to initiate relationships with patients prior to discharge.

> After listening to the news, [the commissioner] merely lit his cigar, leaned back, and said nothing. So his visitors added that for aged patients included in the experimental group, their scores on the Minnesota Multi-

phasic Personality Inventory scale reflecting depression had dropped significantly—again to a statistically significant degree. Even with this exciting contribution, the commissioner remained unimpressed. He had a few questions to ask. They were essentially as follows, but the order was a bit different:

"In your project, you used experienced M.S.W. psychiatric social workers and public health nurses with master's degrees. How do I know that our county welfare workers will be able to match the skills of your project workers? How will we pay for the training programs necessary to prepare the county workers to carry out the same aftercare services?

"Where do I find funds to pay for their travel expenses to state hospitals? Who will carry out the work that they will be unable to accomplish while they are spending the required time at the hospital helping the patients prepare for discharge?" (The commissioner was asking about the Ability to produce the resources needed for the change.)

"How will people in our hospital social service department feel about county workers coming in and taking over a major portion of what they have seen as their roles? And how will the counties feel about extending the duties of their employees beyond the responsibilities which they normally carry?" (He was concerned with violating the assumed Values of the system.)

"Your findings sound almost too simple and pat. How do you know the results you've obtained did not stem from the high skills of the workers on the project: and how do you know that their caseload of only about six patients in any given time wasn't the determining factor?" (The soundness of the Information was being appropriately questioned.)

"In your project, your workers had their offices in a city very close to the hospital and the locations of the patients after discharge were also fairly close. There aren't too many parts of the state where things are that convenient. Will the plan be feasible?'" (The Circumstances, the commissioner was pointing out, would likely work against the success of the change.)

"The counties aren't going to volunteer to use their scarce resources for added service unless legislative and budget adjustments are made.

The state legislature just met. How will I bridge things throughout the rest of the biennium?" (Timing had not been given consideration.)

"Readmission rates already are respectably low. Who is so critically concerned about the problem that the increased expenditures would be warranted? Of course, I'd like to see readmission made unnecessary even for one patient, but it would help if the legislature, the governor, or at least some groups were concerned enough to back this change." (His point was that the Obligation to change was not all that pressing.)

"The need for social workers in our hospitals would be considerably less. Some may lose their jobs. How will I handle their unhappiness? And the county workers are going to be raising Cain because of the hardships they will have to face, even if compensation is arranged. They'll have to stay away from their families during trips to the hospital, for instance." (The commissioner seemed to be reminding us that Resistances had been overlooked.)

"The results are statistically significant, but will the improvement in the readmission rates be sufficient even to be noticed? Will anyone feel a sense of betterment for having gone along with this proposal?" (The reinforcing reward necessary to sustain successful change, the Yield, admittedly was minimal.) (Davis & Salasin, 1978, pp. 109–110.)

The preceding illustration clearly demonstrates the desirability of close collaboration among researchers, practitioners, administrators, and policy makers. In mental health, two of the critical entities in this desired collaboration are the state university and the state mental health authority. The university plays a critical role in research, preservice and continuing education, and technical assistance. The state mental health authority plays an important role in planning, funding, regulating, and operating mental health services. This critical relationship has been recognized in the recent National Institute of Mental Health Public Academic Liaison (PAL) Program (Department of Health and Human Services, 1988).

If the basis of our interest in development of new technology is improvement in the lives of persons with serious mental disorders, then it is clear that the university and the state mental health authority must work closely together. Such a collaboration cannot rely on the old linear transfer model. As an alternative to the linear "knowledge transfer" model, we propose an interactive model of "knowledge exchange" between researchers, practitioners, administrators, and policy makers (similar models have been proposed by others, e.g., Thomas & Robertson, 1990). This type of model envisions a sharing of information between knowledge producers and knowledge users from the initial problem identification stage through the evaluation and adjustment stages. This approach should be to the mutual benefit of researchers, practitioners, and policy makers. The knowledge exchange concept is outlined in five steps.

1. Problem Identification. Conducted jointly by researchers and policy makers or knowledge users; seeks to define issues that require action.
2. Knowledge production. Research that is applicable to resolving the problem; is conducted in such a way that implementation is considered.
3. Policy adoption and implementation. Selection of an application in light of research findings as well as other factors that will best address the issues.
4. Evaluation. Assessment of outcomes to determine if the application had the intended effect.
5. Adjustment. A recognition of the feedback loops. Based on the policy evaluation, the application might require change or modification; or perhaps further research is required; or maybe the original problem requires rethinking or a different conceptual approach.

The above proposed model of knowledge exchange leads to two important logical implications:

1. That the research process itself needs to be expanded on the front end in terms of having more collaborative and developmental approaches to problem identification and selection and on the back end by extending the research process through the period of implementation of research findings.
2. The responsibility for dissemination of research results becomes a much more complex enterprise with a variety of key actors holding different types of responsibility and playing different roles. This requires a much more complex form of accountabilities and requires close collaboration among the parties involved. The foregoing suggests that there is a need for new organizational structures that would tie the research, practice, and public policy enterprises together into ongoing collaborative approaches.

This monograph and much of the research it reports represent the spirit of knowledge exchange, serving as an example of this interactive model. A central theme of many of the chapters in this monograph has been collaboration and information sharing. Research is done in applied settings and is directly applicable to practitioners. There is an effort to avoid jargon, as evidenced by Richard Erikson's terms "remembering things" and "getting around" (Chapter 3 of this volume). While these are laudable efforts, a great deal more work needs to be done to develop these models of collaboration into fully functioning models of knowledge exchange. The remainder of this chapter explores the kinds of questions that must be addressed if the emerging technology of cognitive assessment and treatment is to be of maximum benefit to persons with mental disorders.

Assessing the Readiness of Technology

How do we know if cognitive assessment and treatment technology is ready for dissemination and application?

In trying to answer this question, it is helpful to look at four issues: effectiveness, safety, practicality, and maturity. First, is it effective? To determine whether the technology is effective, we can look at a number of factors such as:

Reliability. Are the results relatively free from error and can they be replicated? Are the same effects evident across multiple trials and settings?

Validity. Do the results actually reflect what we think they reflect; are the results attributable to the interventions? Are the results the product of a scientifically rigorous methodology? For example, did the research employ a good experimental design, a control group, appropriate statistics? (see Cohen, 1980). Is a reasonable case made that we are in fact, measuring or changing that which we proport to measure or change?

Interpretibility. Can we make sense out of the numbers? Are the results unambiguous? Are there clear explanations for the research findings?

Benefit. Do the results indicate that the technology substantially improves the lives of persons served? Will people be better off if this approach is adopted, and how much better off will they be? Are the benefits greater than the risks?

It may be that the question of effectiveness cannot be answered in general, but rather must be discussed in the context of specific populations, particular settings, and identified purposes. For example, many of the chapters in this volume discuss application of cognitive assessment and treatment to persons with schizophrenia, and others have mentioned the application of cognitive assessment to persons with substance abuse problems, organic mental disorders, and affective disorders, as well as stroke victims, the brain-injured, and persons with mental retardation. What other populations can benefit from this technology? Can it be applied to youth with severe emotional disturbances, such as attention deficit disorders?

Many of the discussions have examined the effectiveness of cognitive technology in inpatient settings. But can it be effective in other settings such as outpatient, day rehabilitation, group homes, and in the client's own home? And what about implementation in rural areas? Are there unique barriers to overcome, such as lack of particular types of mental health professionals or access to training, that would limit effectiveness outside metropolitan areas? And for what purpose is the technology to be used? Much of the discussion has focused on application to assessment and treatment, but as discussed in Chapter 4 of this volume, an exciting new purpose that may have potential as well is the area of prevention. Careful examination of the cognitive assessment and treatment technology research presented in this monograph and elsewhere will provide a better idea about what aspects of the technology require further research and what aspects appear to satisfy the question of effectiveness.

SAFETY

A second issue to look at in determining whether a technology is ready is whether it is safe. If the technology is powerful enough to yield positive changes in human behavior and cognition, then there is also the potential to do harm with the technology (Zilbergeld, 1983). We may assume that users of a new and powerful technology will always use it for good purposes. But experiences with past technologies indicate that inappropriate or negligent application can lead to harmful results and violations of individual rights (e.g., Rothman, 1980). Before a technology is ready for widespread dissemination and use, then, we must look at the risk of potential harm: What are the downsides to this technology? Are there people or conditions for which its use is contraindicated? Are there potential iatrogenic effects? For example, there may be potential harm merely in labeling someone as a product of an assessment (Johnson, 1991).

Since all technologies have some potential for harm or misuse, appropriate guidelines and standards must be available before implementation. The first issue is whether existing quality assurance mechanisms are sufficient. For example, if use of the technology is to be confined to particular professions, are the professions' licensure, certification, and regulatory mechanisms adequate to ensure safe application? And is the regulation of the setting in which it is to be applied, as though accreditation or program certification, adequate to ensure safety? Or are some special guidance or regulatory mechanisms required, such as special standards for the delivery of cognitive technologies or for the certification of persons who deliver such technologies?

PRACTICALITY

We have looked at questions regarding the effectiveness and safety of cognitive technology. A third issue to examine in determining if it is ready is whether it is practical. The test of practicality is basically one of resources: time, money, people. The resource questions are always relative. Resources investment must always be judged both in terms of benefit such as cost-effectiveness and in recognition that resources are limited—in other words, to add to something is to take away from something else.

From a time standpoint, one might ask: Is this technology practical in terms of the time it takes to see positive result? Is it reasonable to devote *X* amount of staff time to this? How much time does it take for staff to be trained and to become proficient in the use of the technology? And can service recipients tolerate *X* amount of time per day/month/year devoted to this intervention?

From a cost perspective we might ask: Is this technology practical in terms of overall cost? What are we willing to give up to do this? Can this be substituted for other approaches—in other words, if we do this can we stop doing something else? or is it an additional intervention? Are there potential cost savings from implementation? For example, if a cognitive approach is adopted in a community program, will it lower the probability that an individual will require admission to a more expensive inpatient service? There has been some discussion in this monograph about its capability in preventing relapse. Further, will an inpatient program adopting this approach be able to reduce average length of stay?

From a human resource perspective, there are questions such as those raised by George Hannigan (1991): What kind of and how many people are required to deliver this technology effectively? Are they available? Do people need special credentials such as a Ph.D. in clinical psychology or a graduate degree in occupational therapy to deliver this technology, or can others be trained to do so? And if so, are there minimum qualifications in terms of education and experience? And what are the roles that certain professionals should play in using the technology? For example, what are the roles of psychiatric nurses, social workers, and psychiatrists in applying these techniques? Do people delivering this technology need special backup or access to professional consultation?

And, is the technology practical in terms of capital resources such as space and equipment? What kinds and amount of equipment are required to effectively deliver the technology? What are the physical space requirements? How mobile is the technology? Can it be taken to the person served or must the person come to it? Does it require special space considerations or special computer hardware and software?

MATURITY

A fourth issue is the maturity of a technology. In other words, how far has the technology evolved? In looking at the maturity issue, it is useful to look at three components:

Consensus. Is there reasonable agreement among experts in the field about research results and the application potential of the technology? Is there a reasonable degree of standardization regarding concepts, measurement, intervention strategies, and so on?

Communicability. Is the technology refined to the point that it is easy to understand? Can practitioners and policy makers readily identify application of the research in decision making?

Translatability. Can the constructs and concepts used in the theoretical basis of the technology be translated to meet real-world issues and problems?

In terms of maturity, there is not a bright-line distinction between a mature and an immature technology in most cases. Rather, the evolution of knowledge application can be thought of as a sequence of phases ranging from initial research and development to adoption and application by innovative knowledge consumers to large-scale use by a broader population of knowledge users (see Rogers & Schoemaker, 1971). Generally, however, before a technology achieves broad-based application, the issues of consensus, communicability, and translatability must be worked through.

Dissemination

Once we have determined that the technology is ready—that it is effective, safe, and practical—then it is time to examine the second question: How can or should it be disseminated, promoted, and implemented, and by whom? The central figures in relation to this question are individual practitioners. They are the ones who ultimately put new techniques into practice and who are responsible for its success. This raises four basic questions:

1. Who are the individual practitioners who should be using this technology?
2. What are the prerequisites for their adoption of the technology?
3. Who is capable of influencing these practitioners?
4. How can the practitioners be influenced?

The question of the identity of the practitioners of this technology is important in determining to whom we should direct our implementation efforts. As discussed before, we must decide for whom and in what setting and for what purpose technology is effective, safe, and practical and within that context who should deliver the intervention.

The second issue is prerequisites on the part of the individual practitioner who adopts the new technology. These prerequisites include:

Awareness. The practitioner must know about the existence of the technology.

Understanding. The practitioner must understand the technology and its application.

Motivation. The practitioner must be motivated to use it—for example because the innovation satisfies a need for effective treatment.

Competence. The practitioner must have the knowledge, skills, and abilities necessary to use the technology.

Resources. The practitioner must have the time, equipment, space, and staff support necessary to implement the technology.

Opportunity. The practitioner must have the opportunity to work with the clients in the settings that are appropriate for using this technology.

Any effort to disseminate and implement the technology must consider these prerequisites if it is to be successful. Failure to attend to all of these factors will reduce the effectiveness of the implementation.

The third and fourth concerns of implementation are the influencers and their ways of influencing. There are a variety of people who are in a position to influence practitioners: professionals, administrators, and policy makers.[1] Professionals can disseminate technology information to one another through a variety of roles. One role is that of the scholar-teacher. In this role professionals may disseminate knowledge through publication in professional journals or books, presentation at professional conferences, instruction at the undergraduate and graduate levels, textbooks or other teaching materials, professional workshops and continuing education, and informal communication, by word of mouth. These forms of technology dissemination are the traditional domain of academicians.

A second role of professionals in dissemination and influence is as entrepreneurs. As Davis (1979) points out, there is generally less profit motive in developing and disseminating technology in mental health than in other business fields. Nevertheless, the potential exists for professionals to treat innova-

1. Another category of persons becoming increasingly important in influencing professional practice is consumers of services and the general public. Service consumers and their families are having more and more influence on practitioners and service agencies and the approaches they employ in assessment, treatment, and rehabilitation. These individuals demand procedures that are safe and of demonstrated effectiveness. The general public also demands that services funded through the tax dollar be effective and at the same time cost-efficient. In other words, they want services that work, but they also want those services to be provided within defined resource constraints. An example of the power of citizen advocacy is the public demands on behalf of persons with mental retardation or mental illness when information about the dismal condition of large public facilities came to light in the 1960s and 1970s (e.g., Blatt, 1976).

tions as products to be marketed. For example, a professional might develop and copyright a cognitive assessment instrument or computer software to aid in cognitive assessment and treatment (e.g., IBM Thinkable software). These products could then be marketed to possible users of the technology. The free market approach to diffusion of innovation requires mastering modern marketing techniques—identifying prospective technology users and buyers, identifying the benefits to the buyer of innovation acquisition, and packaging the technology in a way in which the benefits become obvious to the buyer (see Dakin & Lindsey, 1991).

Whereas the first mechanism for dissemination involves professionals talking to other professional colleagues, the second mechanism involves administrators influencing or coercing professionals (see Rogers & Shoemaker, 1971; Glaser, Abelson, & Garrison, 1983). Employers such as hospitals, clinics, mental health centers, community support programs, and rehabilitation agencies can promote innovative interventions by adopting them as part of programmatic or service approaches and by providing employees training to implement the technology. Promotion by administrators may be specific (e.g., an administrator may believe that cognitive treatment and assessment technology should be implemented in a facility), or the promotion may be more general (e.g., the administrator may favor any technology that produces identified outcomes such as improved quality of life, shorter lengths of stay, etc.; to the extent that cognitive technology meets these goals, it will gain favor with administration). The implementation of cognitive treatment techniques and other effective technologies takes place through the strategic decision-making process (see Sethi, Movesian, & Hickey, 1985). The adoption of the innovations can be established as an organizational objective or as a strategy for achieving an objective (e.g., improving the lives of persons served).

Assuming that the administrator has determined the technology to be effective and safe, and that the agency has the necessary resources to apply the techniques to an identified population for a specified purpose, methods for implementation come to the forefront. Implementation will obviously be easier if front-line professions and other direct-care staff are already proponents of the technology. A major challenge for the administrator is accounting for potentially resistant attitudes of professionals who may have used alternative approaches for years. The new technology may conflict with closely held paradigms regarding how assessment and treatment should be administered. This potential resistance may be addressed through modern quality management techniques that involve staff in problem solving and that focus on outcome measures as an objective gauge of change (Leebov & Scott, 1990; Marzalek-Gaucher & Coffey, 1990).

Policy makers, a third group that can influence technology use, are found in legislatures, courts, and the executive branch. Legislators have played an active role in the development of mental health policy over the years. For example, state legislatures generally define the process for civilly committing mentally ill and dangerous persons, create organizational structures for the development of mental health services, and provide statutory safeguards, such as confidentiality protections, for persons who use services (see DeKraai & Sales, 1984).

Generally, legislation is appropriate for developing general responsibilities or for facilitating the development of broad types of service categories such as rehabilitation services, but it is not an ideal forum for implementing a relatively fast-paced, developing technology, primarily because legislation is difficult to change.

Courts have also become involved in social policy development, especially in the last two decades (see Losen, 1977). Perhaps the most prominent examples in the mental health and developmental disabilities fields are the deinstitutionalization cases such as Willowbrook and Pennhurst. The objectives in these lawsuits have been to improve institutional conditions, reduce institutional populations, and develop alternative community services. In some of these cases implementation decrees have specified detailed requirements for staffing ratios, types of staff, and particular assessment, treatment planning, and interventions to be implemented (Note, 1975). However, courts have found such specific standards difficult to implement, and there is considerable controversy regarding the role of courts in administering these policies (Chayes, 1976; Fluckiger, 1985). Furthermore, judicial policy making, at least in the area of service reform, applies only in situations where services fall below the level of minimum constitutional or statutory standards. Policy development by courts, then, is limited to situations where current interventions are substantially deficient (e.g., individual rights are violated) and is not available generally in situations where we might be doing an adequate job but where the policy issue is how we can do the job better.

The third entity responsible for public policy consists of administrative agencies within the executive branch. Generally, within the public policy domain, it is these agencies that are the most common promoters of technological knowledge. If there is agreement that some technology should be adopted throughout the mental health system, there are a variety of options for implementation.

One option is a leadership and planning role; the agency might promote a technology by sponsoring conferences or by recognizing the value of the technology through public planning documents. The goal of a leadership approach is to facilitate the dissemination of knowledge in the hope that mental health professionals and administrators will adopt the technology.

A second public policy option is influence through regulating and accrediting entities. Most public agencies with regulatory and quality assurance responsibilities in human services tend to focus on ensuring that programs meet certain input standards such as levels and qualifications of staff (Human Services Research Institute, 1984).

Often, however, public regulatory agencies are reluctant to impose process standards specifying particular services techniques. It is generally assumed that if the input standards ensure that staff have adequate training, then the professional is in the best position to select from competing approaches the assessment and treatment techniques to be adopted. One of the problems with process standards is that qualifications and training of the regulators must be considerably higher than required for input standards. For example, with cognitive assessment and treatment, regulators would need to have extension knowledge about these technologies, to monitor their implementation. For this reason, process standards are often monitored by professional organizations or national accreditation agencies rather than public agencies.

One way for a regulatory agency to promote a specific technology might be through outcome standards, which relate to the results of services. If a certain technology produces positive outcomes, then a mental health program that adopts the technology is more likely to meet minimum outcome standards than a program not adopting the technology. In this way, programs are not told how to operate services, but rather are provided an incentive to adopt the most efficacious technologies.

A third public policy option for influencing professionals is control of public funding. Funding is an implementation option often tied to a quality assurance and regulatory component. In other words, programs that do not meet regulatory standards are precluded from receiving funds. But funding can be used to promote a technology in other ways as well. For example, an agency may develop standard service categories designating the types of services and components within those services that the agency will fund (Smith & Aderman, 1987). The agency, for instance, might have a reimbursable service category entitled assessment and might require a cognitive component as part of this service.

Another way to promote a particular technology through funding is cost modeling. This approach requires a funding agency to determine the costs of implementing a particular technology—for example, the staffing levels, staff qualifications, facility requirements, hardware such as computer needs—and then to set the maximum reimbursement rate in accordance with these projected costs. Providers then have an incentive to adopt the desired approach because an approach with a higher cost will not be fully reimbursed. On the other hand, if they adopt an approach with a lower cost, they will not receive the maximum level of reimbursement to which they would be entitled for the service.

In looking at these influencers and how they influence, it is evident that there are two broad categories of influence: inducements and requirements. The two are not mutually exclusive and there is usually a mixture of them in any attempt to influence. The challenge is providing a balance appropriate to the issue at hand; in this case, the adoption of cognitive technology. There is, however, a basic public policy question here: To what extent should government and other entities such as third-party payers and accreditation entities seek to influence the practice of individual professionals and their use of particular technologies? Specifically, what should be the role of government and others in promoting or mandating cognitive technologies?

Survey Results

To assist in answering some of the questions raised concerning implementation of cognitive treatment and assessment, a survey was sent to 165 professionals who attended the Cognitive Mental Health Treatment and Assessment Conference held in Lincoln, Nebraska, in February 1991. Twenty-nine of them completed and returned the surveys.

Of the 29 respondents, 3 were researchers, 6 were administrators, 17 were clinicians, and 3 spent half their time in administration and half in clinical work. Ten were from the field of psychology or counseling psychology, eight from occupational therapy, three from recreation therapy, two from social work, and six from other disciplines. The majority of respondents worked in inpatient settings, although 10 respondents worked, at least part of their time, in outpatient, day, residential settings. Twenty-four of the 26 administrators and clinicians worked with persons with affective disorders, eight worked with persons with substance abuse problems, six worked with persons with organic brain syndrome, four worked with youth with severe emotional disturbances, three worked with persons with personality disorders, two worked with persons with brain injuries, and two worked with persons with mental retardation.

Eighty-three percent of the administrator-clinical respondents reported that they used cognitive assessment in their practice or agency, and 78 percent reported that they used cognitive treatment. Many of the respondents, however, qualified their responses by stating that they use cognitive treatment and assessment informally or on a nonroutine basis. Some respondents reporting that they employed this technology used a broad concept of cognitive treatment that included cognitive therapies such as Rational Emotive Therapy. It is clear that the large majority of respondents consider themselves users of cognitive assessment and treatment approaches; however, the level of use and the types of activities they consider to be part of this technology vary substantially.

Respondents listed a variety of potential benefits from cognitive treatment and assessment methods. Many of the identified benefits pertained to improvement in the lives of persons served (e.g., improved cognitive functioning, improved ability to benefit from rehabilitation and skills training, potential for clients to be more successful and productive, improved ability for persons to gain control of their lives and cope with everyday stressors, and potential for a greater sense of accomplishment and improved self-esteem).

Some of the identified benefits pertained to an improved capability of staff to treat disorders (e.g., greater ability of staff to understand the problem, more data for staff to discuss, improved strategies and more specific treatment recommendations, shift in clinicians' thinking, from symptoms to functions, and identification of the titration of medication). Many of the benefits identified by the respondents concern improved capacity for measurement (e.g., more accurate measure of needs and lost ability, measurable outcomes, and monitoring of treatment effectiveness). Finally, some respondents identified changes in consumer placements as a potential benefit of cognitive treatment and assessment (e.g., potential for discharge placements, improved independent living potential, identification of proper placement, prevention potential indicated by reduced likelihood of relapse, increased time away from hospital, and long-term cost savings).

Although the respondents generally agree that there are significant benefits from implementation of cognitive treatment and assessment, they also identified numerous potential barriers to its application. Some of the identified barriers pertained to the cognitive technology itself: the model for cognitive interventions in mental health is still emerging; there is an absence of a unifying theory; it is more difficult and complex than working with overt behavior; there is a limited data base for making decisions about measures and methods of intervention; there are too many unknowns that require additional research; there is a danger of premature hopefulness for untested methods.

Other barriers concerned the training of and acceptance by professionals and staff necessary to implement cognitive techniques (e.g., lack of professional staff in the area; lack of training for staff regarding how to use it and why it should be used; lack of staff coordination and consistency across program areas in implementing the technology; conflict between the cognitive approach and the medical model; lack of general acceptance and possible active resistance by psychiatry; not popular as a form of treatment).

Many respondents identified the human and fiscal resources required to implement the technology as barriers (e.g., more staff is required for interactions, so higher staffing ratios are needed; the application is time-consuming, so it requires additional staff; the staff required to apply the technology is expensive; training materials are expensive; computer applications are expensive).

Other potential barriers identified by the respondents included the following: administrative support is lacking; for successful application, considerable control is needed over the treatment environment; even if the technology is successful in preparing hospitalized patients for community integration, it is difficult to place persons in appropriate community programs; the technology does not apply to all disorders (e.g., obsessive/compulsive); patients may be resistant to using some of the techniques (e.g., leather lacing); patients have difficulty retaining skills learned.

Respondents were split about whether there are potential harms associated with cognitive assessment and treatment. Fifteen thought there were no potential harms, eight respondents thought there were potential harms, and six responded that they did not know whether there were potential harms. The eight persons responding "yes" to this question identified a variety of potential harms. Some of these harms concerned misuse of the technology, as shown in the following responses: there is a danger if it is improperly used or used by persons who are not skilled or qualified to use or interpret the results; there is a danger of overinterpretation on the basis of trivial tasks; there is a danger of neglecting relationship factors when applying techniques; there is a danger in premature use of data to label risk factors in "normals" when actual pathology is absent (e.g., healthy siblings should not be mislabeled); the technology is not yet sophisticated enough to identify heightened genetic risk.

Other potential dangers identified by the respondents included the following: the technology may falsely raise hopes before efficacy data is obtained; these techniques should not be used to the exclusion of other approaches; time and money may be invested in teaching splinter skills that do not generalize to community living; the technology may violate individual rights.

Respondents were asked to state their preferences regarding the mechanism for promoting or encouraging cognitive treatment and assessment technology. Table 10.1 shows these preferences.

Promotion by service agencies and promotion through professional organizations, conferences, and journals were the options most preferred, with graduate level research and training close behind. The public policy–oriented options, and those most likely to be coercive in nature, were least preferred as mechanisms for promoting cognitive mental health innovations. In addition to the options listed on the survey, one respondent identified consumers and families as being important for the promotion of the technology.

In summary, the respondents indicated that cognitive assessment and treatment has the potential to benefit the lives of persons with mental illness.

Table 10.1: Preferred Options for Promoting Cognitive Methods

Option	*Percent of Survey Respondents Choosing Option (n = 29)*
Professional organizations, conferences, journals	93%
Graduate level training or research	86%
Professional certification and licensure	66%
Service agency training and promotion	93%
Program certification and accreditation	69%

Nevertheless, there were a number of barriers identified to using this technology, such as lack of trained staff, lack of research, and a shortage of resources for implementation. Most respondents saw no potential dangers in using the technology; however, some respondents expressed concerns about misuse of the techniques or use of cognitive technology to the exclusion of other approaches. Finally, the respondents expressed a preference for professional universities and service agencies as the primary entities for promoting the technology, rather than government requirements.

Conclusion

While the purpose of this chapter is to raise some important issues related to implementation of cognitive technologies more than to propose definitive solutions to these issues, some preliminary conclusions can be made. Although a complete literature analysis of cognitive treatment efficacy was beyond the scope of this chapter, the research presented in this monograph indicates that cognitive assessment and treatment certainly have the potential for identifying and remediating cognitive deficits in a variety of disabling conditions. It seems likely then that this remediation will positively impact individuals' social functioning, thereby improving the quality of their lives. While further research is needed, these conclusions appear reasonable at this point in time. The survey respondents overwhelmingly agree with this conclusion.

Despite the majority view of the respondents that cognitive technology entails no potential harms, it seems obvious that possible dangers exist with any mental health approach, cognitive technology being no exception. Although the potential harms are not as great as in more intrusive types of interventions such as aversive therapies, psychosurgery, and chemotherapy, possible drawbacks do exist (e.g., misuse of the technology by unskilled professionals or through techniques which are later found to be ineffective, thereby resulting in nonimprovement (or less improvement than after other techniques or after application by competent professionals) of a recipient's quality of life. It seems clear, then, that efforts must be made to ensure that professionals are knowledgeable about the efficacy of varying cognitive assessment and treatment approaches and skilled in application of effective techniques. The effort to ensure application by competent professionals is a joint responsibility shared by universities as primary training forums; professional licensures/certification bodies, which ensure that professionals demonstrate a required level of competence; regulatory authorities, which ensure that provider agencies have met necessary staffing and process standards; and the provider agencies themselves, which have the responsibility for hiring, ongoing staff training, and other internal policy promoting highly skilled professionals.

It is evident, both to the survey respondents and to us, that the promotion of cognitive assessment and treatment technology is primarily the responsibility of service provider agencies, professional organizations, and academia. Regulatory bodies have a lesser role at this level of mental health intervention; however, it should be noted that the majority of survey respondents felt that accreditation-certification-licensure entities had some role in technology promotion, furthering the idea that knowledge dissemination is a collaborative endeavor involving multiple parties. The task becomes, then, not only determining how each entity can most effectively be used to promote cognitive technology (e.g., improved graduate training, sophistication in promoting effective interventions through contemporary management structures), but also how all the entities can be integrated in a comprehensive approach to improve the lives of service recipients. Through the concept of knowledge exchange, all persons concerned about mental health consumers have an important interactive role in problem identification, the knowledge production process, policy adoption and implementation, and evaluation and adjustment of the policies designed to promote this promising technology.

References

Blatt, B. (1976). Purgatory. In M. Rosen, G. R. Clark, & M. S. Kivity (Eds.). *The history of mental retardation: Collected papers,* Vol. 2. Baltimore: University Park Press.

Chayes, A. (1976). The role of the judge in public law litigation. *Harvard Law Review,* 89, 1281–1316.

Cohen, L. H. (1980). Methodological prerequisites for psychotherapy outcome research. *Knowledge: Creation, Diffusion, Utilization,* 2, 263–272.

Dakin, K. J., & S. Lindsey, J. (1991). *Technology transfer: Financing and commercializing the high tech product or service: From research to roll out.* Chicago: Probus Publishing Company.

Davis, H. R. (1979). Change and innovation. In S. Feldman (Ed.), *The administration of mental health services.* Springfield, Ill.: Charles C. Thomas.

Davis H. R., & Salasin, S. E. (1978). Strengthening the contribution of social R&D to policy making. In L. E. Lynn, Jr. (Ed.), *Knowledge and policy: The uncertain connection.* Washington, D.C.: National Academy of Sciences.

DeKraai, M. B., & S. Sales, B. D. (1984). Confidential communications of psychotherapists. *Psychotherapy,* 21, 293–318.

Department of Health and Human Services; Public Health Service; Alcohol, Drug Abuse, and Mental Health Administration, National Institute of Mental Health (1988, September). Announcement: Public-academic liaison (PAL) for research on serious mental disorders (catalog of Federal Domestic Assistance 13.242).

Fluckiger, S. L. (1985). The changing relationship of the judiciary to the policy and administrative processes of governments: An overview of recent commentary on the nature, causes, consequences, and proposals for reform of contemporary judicial encroachment. *Brigham Young University Law Review,* 1985, 671–743.

Glaser, E. M., Abelson, H. H., & Garrison, K. N. (1983). *Putting knowledge to use: Facilitating the diffusion of knowledge and the implementation of planned change.* San Francisco: Jossey-Bass Publishers.

Hannigan, G. (1991). Discussion of papers on mental health administration. Conference on cognitive technology in psychiatric rehabilitation. Lincoln, NE. February 21, 1991.

Human Services Research Institute (1984). *Assessing and enhancing the quality of services: A guide for the human services field.* Boston: HSRI.

Leebov, E. S., & Scott, G. (1990). *Health care managers in transition.* San Francisco: Jossey-Bass.

Marszalek-Gaucher, E. S., & Coffey, R. J. (1990). *Transforming health care organizations: How to achieve and sustain organizational excellence.* San Francisco: Jossey-Bass.

Note (1975). The Wyatt case: Implementation of a judicial decree ordering institutional change. *Yale Law Journal,* 84, 1338–1379.

Rogers, E. M., & Shoemaker, F. F. (1971). *Communication of innovations: Across cultural approach.* New York: The Free Press.

Rosen, P. L. (1977). Social science and judicial policy making. In C. H. Weiss (Ed.), *Using social research in public policy making.* Lexington, Mass., Lexington Books.

Rothman, D. J. (1980). *Conscience and convenience: The asylum and its alternatives in progressive America.* Boston: Little, Brown.

Sethi, N. K., Movsevian, B., & Hickey, K. D. (1985). Can technology be managed strategically? *Long Range Planning,* 18(4), 89–100.

Smith, G., & Aderman, S. (1987). *Paying for services.* Alexandria, Va.: National Association of State Mental Retardation Program Directors, Inc.

Thomas, D. R., & Robertson, N. R. (1990). A conceptual framework for the analysis of social policies. *Journal of Community Psychology, 18,* 194–198.

Zaltman, G. (1979). Knowledge utilization as planned social change. *Knowledge: Creation, diffusion, utilization,* 1, 82–105.

Zilbergeld, B. (1983). *The shrinking of America: Myths of psychological change.* Boston: Little, Brown and Company.

• 11 •

The Story of Cognitive Rehabilitation

Peter A. Magaro

This volume on cognitive rehabilitation (CR) can be read as a play within a play. On the surface it is a remake of a popular drama that reveals a relatively new method to assess and treat mental illness. The play is worth reading because it introduces two actors who starred in the original version of the play and are now creating the same roles in a contemporary interpretation, somewhat like Romeo and Juliet updated into *West Side Story*. Two disciplines, psychology and occupational therapy, are the two actors trying on new roles. Even though they have played the roles in the past, they have never played opposite one another and, in fact, knew of each other only by reputation. The psychologist's prior roles were usually in social farces written by B. F. Skinner that were popular in the academy. The occupational therapist (OT) played the nitty-gritty roles in *One Flew over the Cuckoo's Nest* and other works that involved hands-on experience with patients. Because of their distinct theoretical heritages, they harbor different interpretations of their roles in the new play. The psychologist talks about character development with a mind-set filled with a psychological model that viewed cognitive rehabilitation in social learning terms. The OT views the play from the vantage point of a medical model carried over from working with neurological disorders, with manipulations of the patient intended to change neurological structure.

This volume heralds the double billing of the two professions in a new discipline. A common theory of mental disorders is being forged to champion the therapeutic procedures that define cognitive rehabilitation. The play within the play is a conception of mental illness that is not psychological in the social-cognitive or learning sense, nor is it medical. The role of cognitive processes has given this play its box office appeal and consequent public funding of CR programs. Simply put, the social force that promotes CR is the idea that intelligence is the defining characteristic of the individual, and that the cognitive structures that comprise intelligence can be modified as a computer's programs can be modified. In some cases, the modification is even done by an actual computer.

The introduction of the computer into rehabilitation is not a new wrinkle that makes the job a little quicker and more effective, somewhat like substituting a word processor for a typewriter. The computer as treater is not simply a labor-saving device, an electronic OT worker playing the role of the mental disease terminator. The computer in CR is a manifestation of a popular concept of the person and of mental disorders. The computer is the new model of the person as a cognitive processor, and when the cognitive processing goes awry, it becomes a model of mental illness. While CR derives from theory, the model of behavior is the computer. The computer in CR is therefore not only the dominant treatment tool but also the model of the person: the instrument that mimics thought.

The story I would like to tell concerns the forces in society that have sanctioned the emerging cultural conception of the person as a thinking machine. A consequence of this line of inquiry will be an explication of the theory and the model that give CR its form as a unique treatment method. As such, what does CR mean, i.e., what is the theory behind the treatment? What is its history? How do we conceive of the person in CR? What forces in society share these beliefs and are demanding the establishment of a CR treatment approach? Who in the society is so enthralled with a CR approach to treatment that they will enthusiastically support it?

The Theory, the Model, and Cognitive Rehabilitation

Let me begin by defining some terms: theory, model, information technology, artificial intelligence, information processing, and cognitive rehabilitation itself. A theory is a body of knowledge, ruled by logic, that provides postulates and hypotheses validated by the experimental method. A model is a visible expression of the theory that can be applied to various situations. Models are most useful when the postulates of a theory cannot be directly observed, as in speaking of billiard balls hitting and careening in specific directions to explain the properties of electrons.

Distinguishing between a theory and a model is especially relevant to CR because many occupational and activity therapy treatments are justified by a medical model rather than medical theory. A medical theory contains the body of knowledge that explains physical disease. Infectious and systemic diseases are empirically explained by organ dysfunction or parasitic invasion and are well supported by empirical investigation. The medical theory of physical illness sired a model of mental disorders that has been used to develop hypotheses about the determinants of mental disorders. However, there is no medical theory of mental disorders that has been empirically supported. There are many hypotheses within a unified concept of an illness, but the empirical base needed to give the theory credibility is lacking.

An example of the transformation of a substantiated medical theory into a medical model of mental disorders is the theory of neural dysfunction in Parkinson's Disease used as a model of schizophrenia. Serotonin is necessary for synapse transmission, and a depletion of this substance has been empirically demonstrated to be a causal factor in Parkinson's Disease. A similarity in symptomatology, such as memory loss in both Parkinson's Disease and schizophrenia, encourages the application of the theory of neural transmission to explain schizophrenia in terms of a serotonin deficiency hypothesis. The assumption is that the same neurological process found in the physical disease is also responsible for the mental disorder. However, when the correlates of a serotonin deficiency are empirically examined in schizophrenia, the results are negative. Thus, even though evidence of a physical agent in mental disorders, ranging from brain stem lesions to dopamine dysregulation, has been sought for centuries (every new discovery in medical theory has led to a new explanation of mental illness), no medical theory of mental illness has generated empirical support over time. It remains a model, explaining the possibilities if a medical theory were applied.

Occupational therapists earned their credits in treating neurological disorders within a medical theory and subsequently transferred those procedures to mental patients within a medical model. It is not the model of choice for CR. The danger of adhering to such a model is that it places CR in the role of an auxiliary treatment at most, an indirect way of modifying a neurological structure or chemical process. By implication, treatment methods that directly affect physical structure, such as psychotropic drugs, must remain the primary treatment. A greater problem is that belief in a physical disease will limit the effectiveness of CR because the administration of medication inhibits the cognitive processes being modified. CR does depend upon a theory to justify its use. However, instead of the medical theory, an information-processing theory is required.

Information technoloqy (IT) is the application of computers and the principles of computer science to concrete problems. The major applications of IT rely on the vast electronic storage of information and the reliable response to established cues. IT may range from word processing to tracking missiles. The common element is an orderly progression of decisions that guarantee an identical predictable response to each specific situation. Artificial intelliqence (AI) uses IT to supplant human judgment by simulating human thought. The computer program is a decision-making process that not only stores the vast amount of information required to make decisions in complex situations, but also searches for connections between information bits that allow the most discriminating judgment. While IT is an automation function made possible by the information storage qualities of the computer, AI goes further than most applications by mimicking a form of thinking that retrieves and manipulates information in human form. IT is the obvious manifestation of the information revolution: robots coordinating the operation of steel plants and my use of a word-processing program right now. I cannot think any better by using this machine, but I can write more efficiently. Sections can be deleted, paragraphs can be moved, and words can be correctly spelled. However, I can do the same job with a typewriter or even with a pen—at the cost of a lot more time and effort. Writing with AI, however, would form the nature of this story; the logic would be defined, the organization would follow, and the implications would be drawn. In other words, while the computer helps trains run on time, AI defines the nature of transportation.

An example of rudimentary AI is the programs devised to diagnose mental disorders. The DSM-III criteria are first fed into storage. Two or three experts are then asked to use the diagnostic criteria in the DSM. Use of categories is added wherever the criteria are ambiguous or when multiple decisions have to be made, such as the three or four criteria to be included in making a diagnosis. The computer would store the range of symptoms entered by the evaluator and compare the pattern with the programmed system. The best match of symptom pattern, including steps of exclusion, would produce intelligent diagnostic decisions. A more advanced example of AI would be a chess program that does not rely solely upon the storage of many strategies, but that enters strategies or sequences to be modified immediately in light of the opponent's moves. The computer chess master would learn opponents' moves as a sequence and in its most sophisticated form would categorize the player as a style of chess that can be countered and subsequently defeated.

AI views intelligence as a system of logical epistemology. When an object can be fully described, its function and meaning can be transmitted in the same manner that learning the rules of language can provide some form of speech. The android on *Star Trek,* Lt. Data, is an AI machine. Not only is he programmed with an immense amount of information, but he is also able to think through problems as would humans. The Captain asks him not only to retrieve information but also to analyze the information. He is also able to recognize multiple facial expressions and to draw conclusions about emotions and the interaction of emotion with content to produce different meanings. He is not a simple computer that stores a vast amount of information. He has progressed to the AI stage of a thinking machine, but he is not human. Like his predecessor, the logical Mr. Spock, he can operate only with specific information. He cannot intuit a situation or draw conclusions from vague perceptions. He has the same limitations as AI programs. They cannot operate on the ambiguous no matter how many rules of inclusion and exclusion are stored. For example, a two-year-old child certainly cannot compete with a computer in playing chess or doing arithmetic, but it can recognize its mother's face in a crowd, whereas the computer cannot. The child operates a parallel thought process, while the computer maintains a serial processor, at least at this point in history. Eventually, it is expected that the method of drawing inferences, or recognizing relevant data, or drawing conclusions in the form of scripts will be achieved in AI. (See Dreyfus, 1979; Searle, 1985; or Campbell, 1985 for the debate over the intelligence of computers and the potential of AI).

Information processing (IP) is the theory that defines the cognitive processes that compose thought. It is the theoretical system that AI seeks to imitate to varying degrees of success. The contributions in this volume have used the experimental procedures of cognitive scientists such as Steinberg and Bruner to assess cognitive processes and then to manipulate these processes. Treatment loci would be the encoding process, immediate memory, long-term memory retrieval or storage, or pattern recognition, to name just a few elements of an information-processing system. (See Magaro, 1980, or Magaro, Johnson & Boring, 1986, for a complete description of an information-processing system and its application to treatment.) Enough of the thinking process has been itemized, some would say atomized, to provide treatment of the structure of an IP system.

Cognitive rehabilitation (CR) is the application of IP to the intelligence of mental patients through the use of the computer, which functions as the overt instrument of change as well as the model of change. CR assumes an integrated, interrelated cognitive system that encodes and stores information in multiple forms and that integrates other information into concepts and subsequently into scripts. CR uses the computer to simulate an IP system that when interfaced with a person, can structure the person's thinking process until it operates like the computer. The treatment goal is to mold the cognition of the patient, who is usually schizophrenic, into a sequential processing system that stores relevant information and produces linear logical thought. We do not ask for the creation of novel or unique programs, but only the repetition of thinking that we consider necessary to function in society.

The History of Cognitive Rehabilitation

To understand the history of CR, we must understand the progression of beliefs about the nature of the person. More important, we must understand the nature of the person as idealized at various points in history. This idealization provides the criteria toward which we aspire when as therapists we attempt to "change the person."

Some histories of beliefs about the person are simply lists of the procedures used in treatment of mental disease during a particular era. As such, they are amusing in hindsight, somewhat like laughing at the antics of simple folk, until we realize the suffering that people endured under the guise of treatment. Such history is not enlightening unless it shows why such odd treatment methods were devised. The more informative history of mental disease considers treatment practices in the context of the theory of the mental disease being treated. However, even that is not enough. The most informative history is a history of societal thought. The dominant beliefs in the society instigate theories of madness, and it is these beliefs that must be understood when we inquire why we treat as we do. The emergence of a dominant treatment model follows the popular beliefs about ourselves held by the society. (See Magaro, 1976, for a description of each treatment model and its time, and Magaro, Gripp & McDowell, 1978, for the cultural derivation of a treatment.)

It is thus helpful to consider the dominant contemporary societal beliefs about the nature of the person. As we had Classical man, and then Medieval man, Renaissance man, and Enlightened man, I now introduce Computer man.

This is not the first time that mental health treaters have applied cognitive concepts to treatment. Possibly the period with the clearest template for a cognitive therapy is the interval between 1789 and 1850. It has been called the Age of Individual Worth and the Age of Revolution to celebrate the French revolutions of 1789 and 1848, which bracket the period. The initial revolution of 1789 brought to the culture new political, social, and judicial institutions based upon the principles of individual rights, representative government, and nationalism (Breunig, 1970).

When democracy fell into disarray after the First Republic, Napoleon established order in the form of an enlightened despot praised by Voltaire, Kant, and Goethe. Bernard (1973) welcomed "a sense of reasoned organization pursuing an orderly life." England's revolution, nicely labeled the Silent Revolution by Osborne (1970), took a less tremulous path but resulted in the dominance of the same values applauded in France. Social legislation fueled by the Horatio Alger mythology in the United States reflected a belief in the freedom and responsibility of the individual, who had the intellectual and moral ability to form a binding social contract that would benefit the community. The dominant belief was that, through reason, individuals will devise solutions to social problems. The faith in the responsibilities of the reasonable individual framed a judicial system and liberated repressive institutions. For instance, one of the first acts of the First Revolutionary Government in France was to order all the mad released. Philipe Pinel broke their chains when he contended that being deprived of liberty contributed to madness.

These beliefs flourished in the wealth created by the industrial revolution, which seemed to invent new machines daily. We sometimes forget the number of inventions during this period: Eli Whitney's cotton gin, the steamboat, the locomotive, the submarine, gas lighting, cast steel, and Faraday's electric motor. Social inventions were as frequent: the *Encyclopedia Britannica,* vaccination against smallpox, infrared rays, photographs, the table of atomic weights, morphine, the shrapnel shell, tin cans, vacuum bottling factories, covered bridges, and Colgate-Palmolive soap. The avalanche of products created a large middle class that invested in the huge metal structures to house the first assembly lines.

The standard of life dramatically changed. Average real income doubled during this period in England. Quality and type of foods increased. For the first time in history, meat was a common food for a working family. New industries such as steel and construction produced high-paying labor positions. Time was measured better, buildings were bigger, transportation was faster. A single machine could replace 50 people as steam drove huge engines. It is no wonder that the beliefs of the time were taken as the truths of a just society.

Of interest in the technological revolution is what happened to the mad. Foucault (1965) traces the path of the mad in France as they were transferred to asylums from poorhouses under the guidance of the social conscience evolving at the time. The story of Pinel is most instructive of that period; he instituted a therapy program that qualifies him as the father of cognitive rehabilitation.

Pinel assessed the patient on the basis of cognitive functioning, noting disturbances in attention, memory, and judgment. His treatment was called "moral synthesis," by which he meant education through the senses, and it used three procedures to correct deviant cognitive processes: silence, recognition by mirrors, and perceptual judgment. Silence taught the person to recognize that he or she was projecting a false image; such patients were ignored when they spoke of their delusions. Recognition by mirrors led patients to take note of themselves and how they were acting mad, an olden-day version of the Three Christs of Ypsilanti. In perceptual judgment, Pinel told patients that their conclusions were erroneous and that if they did not change their perceptions, Pinel would do it for them. The patient had no appeal to anyone beyond Pinel. When a patient refused to be reasonable, for example by not eating, Pinel and a muscular staff would come to the door rattling chains and ordering the patient to eat or else.

Benjamin Rush had similar ideas in the United States. He wanted the mad to regain their will, which was defined as fulfilling the social contract. He would shock the patient back to reasonableness by deception, dunking in cold water, or gyrating chains. He was insistent in the belief that he could change a patient's judgment. Obviously, being a mental patient in the nineteenth century was frightening work. I doubt that there was any serious malingering.

Hence, this a school of cognitive therapists believed they could modify thought in terms of both its content and its structure. The world was benefiting from the rational urge. There was no reason not to believe that tuning the intelligence (memory, attention, and judgment) would erase mental problems. Of course, there were those who missed the point and confused the model with the theory. They took the industrial revolution literally. They saw machines build cities, and heard the tremendous advances in medicine at this time, such as Harvey's circulatory theory. From this it took only a short simpleminded step to concoct the formula to rebuild a damaged mechanical mind. Patients were dunked into vats of cold water to contract blood vessels believed to be enlarged by the restricted bile that was inflaming the brain. Blood-letting and transfusions were also applied. However, the most literal interpretation of the technological culture was the eating of iron capsules. Since iron was the main material in building the industrial society's locomotives, huge bridges, and the Glass Palace in London, mental patients were thought to benefit from ingesting iron tablets to strengthen their nerves. The blood vessels were too rigid or too soft. Mixing iron into the blood would provide the proper malleability and consequently free the bile. Soap was also fed to the mad because it was had been found to drastically reduce communicable diseases; hence, a little cleaning out of the mental system would produce a shining, healthy mind.

The goal of all treatments was to return reason to a position of control. Reason was king and distractibility was the sign of a disturbed mind. The sudden shot of a cannon, a quick dunk, would shock the mad out of their reveries or return the flaccid neurological structure to the right stuff of serious reasonable people.

Thus, today is not the first period of CR, nor is it the first time that a society has been enamored of a mechanical mind. Even though cognitive concepts are more refined today and the model is closer to the theory, we are still echoing our treatment ancestors with our faith in the economics of rational thought. Like prior treatment movements, CR will eventually be tested for its effectiveness rather than for its adherence to cultural norms.

If it does not pass this test, it will fade into history as another cognitive procedure that did not work, a quaint program applied to the mad in the service of a conformity to cultural values. The Age of Revolutions propagated treatments in the belief that the reasonable liberated person produced a common good through technology. The societal beliefs of the present foster an IP theory and subsequently CR as the treatment of choice.

The Model Embedded in Contemporary Society

This brief history of the Age of Revolutions illustrates the social forces that created the acceptable treatments of the time. Now let us turn to contemporary society, to identify the social engines that are thrusting treatment into a computer model. Basically, CR is "hot" today because our society, in the grip of IT, believes people act as they do because of the manner in which they process information.

Consider the tools that define our experience of reality. Begin with Lewis Mumford's (1934) statement that the invention of the clock made a deeper impact on human experience than the invention of the printing press. Print certainly introduced and disseminated ideas as well as producing a consensual history, but the clock altered at a deeper level the way the world is experienced. Print was an "enabling technology" with which we could do familiar things more effectively, but the clock was a "defining technology" because it caused an experiential paradigm shift. Our place in time was shifted from the passive long-term orientation to the active short term. We now could manage time and with it our mode of production. For instance, in the fabrication industry, clocks standardize motion by allocating the units of time required for automation (Solomonides and Levidow, 1985).

The computer is a technology that defines effective thought, a serial connected thinking within a massive storage capacity that ignores not only emotions but also intuition and disconnected associations. We demand serial sequential thought with full memory of past target events and those related to them. Other types of thinking such as the inductive or the intuitive or the inspirational are not at the same level of acceptability. The computer has relegated such thought to the frivolous or, at the most, the artistic. What has raised the computer to such exalted heights that it prescribes the correct mode of thought?

We love the computer and imitate its thinking because we are long down the road of a technological society. The occupational fate of individuals as well as the fate of nations depends upon technological prowess; thus it is not surprising that the computer and its inherent thinking process is idealized to the same degree as personal responsibility and iron in the nineteenth century. It is a given, like the air we breathe, that a superior technology is the only way to turn a profit in contemporary capitalistic economic systems. "Once the principle is accepted that something ought to be done because it is technically possible to do it, all other values are dethroned, and technological development becomes the foundation of ethics" (Reich, 1970, p. 34).

The owner of the most efficient system will be the one who succeeds; in other words, labor is machine-dependent. However, when we speak about person-machine dependency we are no longer thinking about making machines more user-friendly. The interest in automation has gone beyond the release of the person from menial labor and assembly-line production to placing the person in the context of a labor system where his or her thinking processes can be manipulated to increase production. The Japanese excel at this practice. Performance on the line is closely tied to the individual's self-worth as constantly monitored by the industrial output of the individual's team. The belief is that the individual's performance can be manipulated by managing the cognitive constructs that refer to the self-image, and that these constructs can be established by management and maintained by the peer social environment. The person is thought of as a tuneable machine. As one can modulate sound on a stereo, the output of the worker also can be adjusted to play the tune exactly. When the tuning is correct, all that is necessary is posting a diagram for each task that presents in minute detail the actions required to maintain the most efficient production, along with a manager who will continually evaluate work performance and feed back the results to the worker.

Like the Romantics in the Age of Revolutions, some rebel against such a manipulated, sterile existence. Some feel they are being judged under a harsh technological light that is not flattering to their personality. For instance, imagine that two women apply for a job as a checkout person in a supermarket. Mary has little experience with machines and a fear of computers; however, she is friendly and describes herself as a "people person." The other candidate, Joan, describes herself as a serious person who likes schedules and keeping things in order, and although not familiar with computers, she would like to learn how to operate them. Joan is hired. Even though the store prides itself on having "the friendliest staff in town," they want Joan because the job description prioritizes the operation of a computerized checkout system. Management wants to find people who are sequential in their thinking, are more efficient, mesh better with the checkout machine, than those who enjoy and consequently are distracted by customers.

Hiring people in terms of skills or traits that match job specifications is nothing new. What is not so obvious is how the economic demands of a society create an image of "the desirable individual" in fields ranging from checkout clerk to manager. The checkout search is a concrete example of the manner in which a technological economy selects the few for success. However, more important than the person meshing with a computer is the style of thought that is being idealized: the human thinking machine that is rewarded in our society. The chosen ones of today think like computers.

The world of the therapist is no different from that in any other institution in our society. A particular worldview is required to operate the machines deemed necessary to perform the job. As with Joan and Mary, a new way of checking out the patient is being demanded. The computer not only moves food along the counter more effectively. It also moves a patient through treatment. Some treaters feel that the push for computerized methods dismisses the human touch required in the care of any person. They do not approve of the role of computers as treaters and do not comprehend CR in technological terms. The treatment world is upside down. OT programs are no longer supplementary but the main treatment of mental patients. It is like *Alice in Wonderland*. Physicians are auxiliary treaters, called in to consult on drugs, but they are not the treaters of choice. They are only treaters when an OT is not available, and the OT must be computer-compatible. What is going on?

Briefly, the society demands a therapy that will change the mind, alter the intelligence, of an individual because society believes in IP, at however simple a level. The consensual belief is that a person is composed of cognitive structures that determine the effectiveness of social performance. The simple next step is to apply this belief in the form of a therapy that alters thought processes by means of the technology proven to have exacted technological change, the computer. The society believes in the efficacy of ideas that reside within an electronic person, and, as we have seen, we have always applied to the mental patient the technology of which we are enamored.

As psychoanalysis permeated the 1940s and 1950s, or as humanistic therapies filled the 1960s and behavioral therapies dominated the 1980s, cognitive therapies are taking control of the 1990s. The increasing popularity of CR does not stem solely from scientific evidence of its effectiveness nor from a theory, IP, that can empirically explain a mental disorder. Like prior popular treatment movements, it fulfills a zeitgeist. Contemporary society has defined an ideal that is to be replicated in those who are mad, creating Igor-like practitioners, building the bodies conceived of by HAL, the malicious computer of the movie *2001: A Space Odyssey*. A technological person with modifiable cognitive processes is an idea that has found its time.

However, just saying that the time is ripe for the emergence of the computer person does not say enough. It is more than the economics of a time that advances a particular technology. There has to be a personality of the time who wears the cultural mantle of the favorite luminary. The ideal today is the person who is most computer-like and consequently best suited to manage the amount and specificity of information that is required to operate effectively in any aspect of society. The personality type that will ride the wave of IT is the compulsive. Compulsives will expand their influence in the 1990s because, according to Toffler (1970), the elite will be those who can best manage an information-laden society.

The Compulsive Personality in Society

Society has always idealized a form of thought and has rewarded the prototypes of the thinking style with material success. For instance in the initial stages of the industrial revolution, when the economic power of the bourgeoisie was rapidly accelerating, the worldview honored calculation and rationality as the mainsprings of the economic revolution (Von Martin, 1932). Those who dissented from placing such cognitive processes on a pedestal were called Romantics and were assigned to the art world or to some other misty place where they, like women, "didn't understand this thing called business."

This was not the first time that a cognitive style had been recognized as essential for the betterment of a state. Martines (1963) noted the similarities between the economy of the Renaissance and the type of intellect praised. The Florentines who led society out of the Medieval Age were the professionals and merchants who demanded a rationalistic worldview. They reinvented a world of trade that required a financial medium of exchange involving the skills of abstraction, objectivity, and quantification. Those individuals who could facilitate the exchange of the medium were of immense value and rose to manage the society, eventually expanding their spheres of influence by commissioning the art that promoted their ideals. Those who succumbed to the pull of time and place were cognitively at home in faith and meditation. They could not compete in the rapid maneuver of the trade and consequently were superfluous.

The celebrated art of the Renaissance reflected the values of the capitalists who replaced the nobles and clergy as the leaders of society. Antal (1948) compared the painting of Masaccio and Gentile da Fabriano and found that each appealed to different social classes. Gentile appealed to the feudal audience, which by this time was limited to the old aristocracy and the bishops, while Masaccio appealed to the new upper middle class of the guilds. Masaccio's art is matter-of-fact, sober, and clear-cut. Gentile's is ornate, decorative, and hierarchic. Masaccio became the favorite of the time because he expressed the cognitive worldview.

Jones (1961) and Burke (1974) proved the same point when they discovered the value dimensions in the literature of the Renaissance as compared with the literature preferred by medieval lords and clerics. The Renaissance merchants emphasized natural laws, while the nobles stressed the mysteries of the supernatural. The merchants respected achievement rather than birth, letters rather than arms, action rather than contemplation, will rather than fortune, reason rather than faith, dignity rather than misery, and individualism rather than an adherence to tradition. In short, the rapid social and political change of the Renaissance idealized the person, of whatever social class, who manifested the cognitive style required by the mercantile economy.

Thus, any place in time has a particular idea about the nature of the person and of life, but the dominant idea, which forms the institutions, is that held by the group who holds economic power. Their ideas are objectified and they pronounce the attitudes to be held by the society at large. Returning to the job in checkout, Mary would have been hired in a medieval grocery store. Concern with efficiency would not have been relevant as Mary's friendly (possibly spiritual) manner would have led to her being commended as St. Francisca of the cash register. Joan, however, is hired in our time because she is of our time. Her serial thought mimicks the computer and makes her a smashing checkout android.

Every cultural epoch searches for the person who embodies the spirit of the time and has the skills demanded by the economic nature of the society. Treaters enthusiastically follow the dominant societal worldview because they are part of the society. At present, they believe in habilitating and rehabilitating the cognitions and their model of replication is the person who lives a computer existence, the compulsive personality.

The Compulsive Personality Type can be summarized by describing the cognitions, emotions, and values of the people who express the type. Their cognition has been characterized as precise, deliberate, rational, and capable of great concentration. Graham Reed (1985) has described them as highly single-minded. Memory tends to be sharp and recall is more detailed than in others. With such an emphasis upon precision, it is not surprising that compulsives insist upon accuracy in descriptions, recollections, plans, and instructions. The orderly, meticulous attention to detail appears pedantic, and their judgment has been described as cautious, realistic, and pragmatic. In the extensive amount of clinical descriptions of the compulsive personality, a trait listed by Abraham (1921) is particularly applicable to our discussion: "Pleasure in indexing and classifying . . . the drawing up of programmes and regulating work by time sheets" (Abraham, 1953 [1921] pp.378–388, in Millon, 1981, p.221). With such an emphasis upon precise cognitive functioning and such a joy in wielding the intellect, it is not unexpected that one of the prominent values of the compulsive personality is being rational. Their motto emulates Descartes: "I think, therefore I am." If something has no rational order, it does not exist.

Edward Spranger (1928) in his book *Types of Men* described a personality type called the theoretic. This personality was a thinker, the big planner of life's goals, who wished to be a consistent entity in a world of order. As such, he or she directed all thoughts toward elaborate plans to impose order upon a world that seemed to be in chaos. The ideal was a highly ordered society governed by "a complex set of laws which are interrelated to each other according to strict cognitive legality." The compulsive personality believes that truth is derived from a series of logical deductions organized into a system of knowledge, an epistemology, that creates a standard of belief. Other forms of engendering knowledge are dismissed. Most of us walk a crooked path between self-doubt and revealed truth in adapting to a perplexing society that transmits a babel of messages on how we should act, feel, and want. The compulsive personality steps on the line and firmly resolves the issue.

Another god in the pantheon of the compulsive personality is the prediction of events. Such people demonstrate an overriding need to control most aspects of life. The pervasive desire to predict, to place events and people in categories, is not limited to intellectual matters. The compulsive personality is infamous for a need to construct elaborate schedules, portioning out time to be spent in work and play, to the point where periods of relaxation are performed as a task. In becoming the complete "pocket-planner," placing their lives in order through a folder of dates and times, they manage anxious uncertainty while at the same time promoting a cognitive style of small, orderly thought units.

The Achilles' heel of this protective intellectual order might be thought of as an emotional näiveté, an inability to bring feeling into the world of ideas. Emotionally, compulsives are described as cold, distant, and superrational. The term "isolation of affect" refers to their emotional detachment and insensitivity. In effect, they squeeze the juice of life out of an issue through their insistence upon intellectual distinctions. They do not empathize with the emotional tug-of-wars that fuel political issues, so they ignore them. They prefer to bask in the light of rational understanding, not sullied by irrational feelings.

Most of all, compulsives are different from other personality types in the manner in which they use information. Like the computer, they are driven to form systems of thought. Shapiro (1965) described the cognitive characteristics of the compulsive personality as a thinking process that is sharply focused on the technical or detailed aspects of situations, along with a diminished capacity to switch to impressionistic cognition. The compulsive wards off emotions by focusing on the detailed and technical aspects of the environment. Shapiro argues that this sharply focused attention and intense, directed activity of the compulsive affects decision making, and is, more generally, an experience of reality devoid of emotional shading. Shapiro compares the compulsive to a pilot flying in a dense fog with only instruments as guides. "He can fly as if he were seeing clearly, but nothing in his situation is experienced directly." Shapiro notes that in making a decision the compulsive fares all right if a rule or formula can be applied; however, if the decision requires "going with what you feel," the compulsive will experience great difficulty. Compulsives typically do not ask themselves such questions as "Does it feel right?"; such a question is not relevant to them since "feeling" is not a salient aspect of experience. The questions "Does it fit?" and "Does it meet the specifications?" are more meaningful. Compulsives, therefore, may not be avoiding feeling but may instead be inadvertently eliminating feelings by their means of processing information. The cognitive style of the compulsive encourages a detachment from personal events, what Reed (1985) labels a lack of personalization.

The thinking processes, therefore, serve many useful purposes for the compulsive personality. The processes aid in inhibiting emotions; they promote a sense of autonomy; and they provide a means of control of the self and others. However, while cognitions can be seen as being in the service of motives, a medium to satisfy needs, another interpretation is that the medium is the message. The nature of the compulsive's cognition determines behavior. For instance, when the compulsive is observed searching for more and more information to complete a task, the inference is drawn that he or she is fulfilling a need for control. However, the alternate view is that the cognitive process itself is the mainspring of behavior. Behavior is produced by the cognitive process of systematization. In effect, if a cognitive structure requires a great deal of information in order to function, you fill it up whenever you can. Most of the compulsive's life consequently runs according to a preconceived inviolable program. Any change in the program produces a range of distressful reactions ranging from annoyance to intense anxiety. The preference therefore is to adhere to a plan that enhances clarity. While it is true that such a cognitive style results in the control of people and events, the need in a cognitive sense is to reduce conceptual ambiguity.

It should be clear that the compulsive personality is a normal, well-adjusted individual. Reed (1985) presented the most complete characterization of the compulsive personality and its pathology. He differentiated people who exhibit psychiatric symptoms, such as obsessions or compulsions, from the compulsive personality. "Obsessions" and "compulsions" are terms that describe a temporary symptomatic state that many people experience at one time or another. The term "compulsive" is applied instead to a configuration of traits. Compulsives could also exhibit obsessions or compulsions and in fact would be predisposed to exhibit such symptoms when undergoing stress; however, such symptoms are rare in this day and age. Typically, the compulsive personality trudges along in a normal manner, mastering the world.

The compulsive personality is best suited to a telecommunications society where the system is the message. The compulsive's cognitive and emotional traits mesh well with a complex society that demands specialized knowledge to interface with the technology required to perform tasks from the simplest, such as withdrawing money from a bank through a machine, to the most complex, as in devising an automated assembly line or shooting a rocket to Mars. Consequently, the image of the compulsive personality may be an economic necessity in a technological world.

Paykel and Prusoff (1973) pointed out that the traits of the compulsive personality suggest a "hard-working, ambitious, industrious, consistent, well-controlled, and worthy citizen" (p.317). Pollitt (1960) found such people to be more gifted, intelligent, and energetic than others. Previous authors agree that compulsive traits are highly valued in our society. Kaplan (1987) considers the compulsive character the most prevalent today and its defense mechanisms the most widely utilized.

Pollack (1979) considers compulsive traits to be so valued within a capitalistic technological society that they generate great self-worth and social acceptability. In fact, it has been argued that in Western cultures, the compulsive personality is the most valued social character, embodying the work ethic within a capitalistic social and economic organization (Homigman, 1967). Many of the traits characteristic of the compulsive personality—for example, perseverance, self-control, ambition, autonomy, thriftiness, high need for achievement—are the traits that allow the successful operation of a capitalistic, technological society. The compulsive personality consequently has been observed to prevail in Western and non-Western advanced industrial societies such as that of Japan (Gorer, 1943) but, as would be expected, they are not as prevalent in third world economies or in primitive cultures (Lin, 1967).

Compulsive personality traits are tailor-made for industrialized societies, which require individuals to apply the intellect to control their destiny and conquer the natural world. The compulsive needs to understand and control the self in order to keep the world on a predictable level. The personality characteristics of perfectionism, concern for details, and intellectualization all combine to produce a person capable of the intricate, theoretical, and often tedious work required to master the role of a technocrat or a scientist. While the compulsive as a technocrat or scientist may not be prone to creative, innovative discoveries that require an inductive grasp of relationships, compulsives are able to understand underlying principles that enable them to explore new subject matter and devise solutions. As investigators, they would be valued for the ability to assemble many data pieces into a theoretical system that could explain and solve economic and social problems. They would also display the capability of confirming or rejecting hypothesized solutions, followed up by a painstaking attention to the minute aspects of a particular problem. The compulsive as a scientist, for instance, would feel most at home in the scientific fields that lead to the most definite predictions, such as engineering, physics, and biology. Kokosh (1971) reports that compulsives, in fact, do achieve more in physics and zoology than they do in less precise fields such as sociology and history. On a more tangential level, Termen (1955) found that even at an early age, scientists exhibited an interest in science, and as adults, they scored lower than nonscientists in social relations, preferring solitary activities, being slow in social development and indifferent to close personal relationships, characteristics assigned to the compulsive personality.

Richard Ashbrook and I (Magaro & Ashbrook, 1985) explored the personality of social groups defined by the choices people made regarding leisure or work activities. We tested Protestant religious groups, computer programmers, and medical technologists as well as other professionals such as car salesmen and those participating in recreational activities such as a softball league. When we compared groups on the personality style scales, we found that computer programmers scored higher than all the other personality types on the compulsive personality scale. The medical technologists were second highest. Compulsives are therefore very much in evidence within specific professional groups.

If I may now be permitted a bit of hyperbole, compulsive personalities are everywhere around us. Their personality is a blueprint for success in the elite occupations but more important, they have defined "proper patterns of thought" as modeled on a information-processing system. Their prototype is so powerful that it can be said that we have entered the Age of the Compulsive. Their values echo around us from the theater, the cinema, political campaigns, marketing themes, and mental illness warnings. Their manner of work has become a management standard embodied in the criteria for job advancement. Their style of consumerism has shaped advertising images and their product preferences have become essential to living the good life. Their modes of play have become national crazes, with leisure industries springing up to supply the necessary playthings. Their feeding habits have redefined proper diet, drastically changing the foods certified as edible. The compulsive, in effect, has become the cultural ideal of how we work, play, eat, buy, and dress, and, most important, of what values to hold dear. Their beliefs are so dearly held that they define the standard of American success. Their envoys are the toast of the town, celebrating a lifestyle to the applause of their countrymen. Yes, they are all around you: your hard-working neighbor, your mayor, your trusted colleague, your friend. Being ubiquitous, this personality is the key to understanding the appeal of a particular politician, the imbroglio of corporate culture, and the character of leaders, as well as the devotion of the perpetual jogger and the yuppie lifestyle. They are a small group numerically, but they are the power elite: the blood and guts of American institutions who reek of the scent of status to the point where others lust to imitate their psychological prowess.

The values of the compulsive personality are such a prevailing standard of belief that when they compose a song of themselves, they are singing all-time favorites from the American songbook. For example, how often have you heard praises sung for efficiency and long-term planning? They sound like the skeleton keys that unlock the doors to the good life in any place or time, but those values are not universally shared. Faith in a planned world is nothing more than a hallmark of the compulsive personality projected upon the fabric of society. Members of other cultures often believe we have gone overboard in promoting the values of efficiency and long-term planning. Fate and a few spirits, the mysteries of life; those ambiguous happenstance events that signal the unexpected are the forces that turn the wheel of life.

More important, compulsive personalities go beyond promoting a few slogans on living the good life. They demonstrate how to think and feel in order to live the good life. The compulsive patrimony is not just *what* one should think, but how one should think: the thinking processes that underlie political and social beliefs. For instance, the compulsive personality does not highly value intuition or emotionality. Consequently, social positions tainted by emotional appeals or bolstered by intuitions are discounted. The acceptable view requires a tempering in the cool beam of reason.

Returning to the theater of CR, the real play is the treatment of the compulsive, by the compulsive, for others, namely the mad. We believe we can manage an artificial intelligence system now that we have the tool via the model. We assume that all can think the way of the compulsive, as a living computer, and that this style of thought is a necessity to function in today's technological society. We answer the question of what we want to accomplish by stating an adaption to a technological society. We answer the question of what the patient shall become through our rehabilitation efforts by forming an image of a human computer. We answer the question of our conception of the ideal person or the cured patient as the compulsive personality. We answer the question of the role of CR in society as the cutting edge of the inevitable economic reality. As Pogo would have said, "We seen the future and it is us."

References

Antal, F. (1948). *Florentine painting and its social background.* London: K. Paul.

Bernard, J. F. (1973). *Talleyrand: A biography.* New York: Putnam.

Breunig, C. (1970). *The age of revolution and reaction.* New York: W. W. Norton Inc.

Burke, P. (1974). *Tradition and innovation in Renaissance Italy.* London: Fontana/Collins.

Campbell, J. (1895). *Grammatical man.* New York: Penguin Books.

Dreyfus, H. L. (1979). *What computers can't do.* New York: Harper Colophon.

Foucault, M. (1965). *Madness and civilization.* New York: Mentor Books.

Jones, W. T. (1961). *The Romantic syndrome: toward a new method in cultural anthropology and history of ideas.* The Hague: Nijhoff.

Gorer, G. (1943). Themes in Japanese culture. *Transactions of the New York Academy of Science,* 5: 106–124.

Kaplan, A. H. (1987). Obsessive-compulsive phenomena in adult obsessionality, compulsive personality disorder and obsessive compulsive disorder (neurosis). *Psychiatrty Journal of the University of Ottawa,* 12: 214–221.

Kokosh, J. (1971). Two-point MMPI code types and academic achievement. *Psychological Reports,* 28: 671–676.

Lin, T. (1967). The epidemiological study of mental disorders by WHO, *Social Psychology,* 1: 204–205.

Magaro, P. A. (1976). *The construction of madness: emerging conceptions and interventions.* New York: Pergamon Press.

Magaro, P. A. (1980). *Cognition in schizophrenia and paranoia.* Hillsdale, N. J.: Lawrence Erlbaum Associates, Inc.

Magaro, P. A., & Ashbrook, R.M. (1985). The personality of societal groups. *Journal of Personality and Social Psychology,* 48, 1479–1489.

Magaro, P. A., Gripp, B., & McDowell, D. (1978). *The mental health industry: A cultural phenomenon.* New York: Wiley Interscience.

Magaro, P. A., Johnson, M., & Boring, R. (1986). Information processing approaches to the treatment of schizophrenia. In R. Ingram (Ed.), *Information processing approaches to psychopatholoqy and clinical psycholoqy.* New York: Academic Press.

Martines, L. (1963). *The social world of the Florentine humanists.* Princeton: Princeton University Press.

Millon, T. (1981). *Disorders of personality: DSM III Axis II.* New York: Wiley Interscience.

Mumford, L. (1934). *Technics and civilization.* New York: Harcourt Brace.

Osborne, J. W. (1970). *The silent revolution.* New York: Charles Scribner's Sons.

Paykel, E. S., & Prussoff, B. A. (1973). Relationship between personality dimensions: Neuroticism and extraversion against obsessive, hysterical and oral personality. *British Journal of Social and Clinical Psychology,* 12, 309–318.

Pollack, J. M. (1979). Obsessive-compulsive personality: A review. *Psychological Bulletin,* 86, 225–241.

Pollitt, J. D. (1960). Natural history studies in mental illness: A discussion based on a pilot study of obsessional states. *Journal of Mental Science,* 106, 93–113.

Reed, G. F. (1985). *Obsessional experience and compulsive behavior.* Orlando, Fla.: Academic Press.

Reich, C. A. (1970). *The greening of America.* New York: Random House.

Roe, A. (1953). *The making of a scientist.* New York: Dodd, Mead.

Searle, J. (1985). *Minds, brains and machines.* London: BBC Publications.

Shapiro, D. (1965). *Neurotic styles.* New York: Basic Books.

Simmon, W. E., Primavera, L. H., Klein, B., & Cristal, R. C. (1972). Personality and nonverbal rigidity: Some preliminary findings. *Journal of Psychology,* 82, 127–132.

Solomonides, T., & Levidow, L. (1985). *Compulsive technology: computers as culture.* London: Free Association Books.

Spranger, E. (1928). *Types of men.* Halle: Max Neimeyer Verlag.

Terman, L. M. (1955). Are scientists different? *Scientific American* Reprint, January, 3–7.

Toffler, A. (1970). *Future shock.* New York: Random House.

von Martin, A. (1944). *Sociology of the Renaissance.* London: Harper Torchbooks.

• 12 •

Cognitive Technology in Psychiatric Rehabilitation: A Town Meeting

Mary Sullivan

The discussions this chapter describes took place at a conference designed to stimulate and facilitate interaction between researchers, clinicians, and mental health administrators. Originally a small gathering was anticipated. It was hoped that people of related scientific and professional backgrounds would challenge and be challenged by each other in a manner customary in professional and scientific conferences. However, because the response of regional clinicians and others to the conference invitation was so much greater than expected, discussion was enhanced by a more far-ranging and inclusive introduction of ideas and perspectives. It became a "town meeting" of a fairly large and diverse professional and consumer community.

As with all successful professional conferences, more questions were raised than answered. As with all successful town meetings, participants staked special claims to various issues, so that both conflicts and common ground were discovered and explored.

The format of the conference included four formal discussion panels, each panel strategically placed on the program to facilitate discussion of topically organized presentations. The presentations were preliminary versions of many of the chapters in this book. The role of the panelists was vital in the town meeting process, their comments serving to inspire and enhance subsequent questions and open discussion with the audience (the identities of the panelists, to whom all the conferees owe a significant debt of gratitude, are listed in the Acknowledgements of this volume). As might be expected, the themes that emerged across the entire town meeting transcended the original topical organization of the conference. In retrospect (actually, after much subsequent review of and reflection upon videotapes of the entire proceedings), four major themes coalesced: the importance of clinical assessment, the nature of mental health systems, ethical issues, and professional and training issues. This account addresses in turn the exchange of ideas that occurred with regard to each of these themes.

Clinical Assessment

The role and the value of assessment were stated several times, in various ways. In rehabilitation, assessments are essential in shedding light on the individual's strengths as well as on problems or disabilities. Assessment should address all aspects of personal and social functioning, from molecular to molar levels of analysis. Because assessments need to be comprehensive, the assessment team should be interdisciplinary. No one professional group has the proverbial corner on the assessment market. This appears to be as true for the special case of cognitive assessment as for clinical assessment in general. Even within the cognitive domain, there is a significant range of interest, from the molecular processes of attention and memory to the more molar processes of conceptualization and social problem solving. At this time, there is no single technology or approach that comprehensively addresses all the cognitive levels in an integrated manner.

In rehabilitation, assessments should be used in several ways, not solely as a one-time diagnostic event at the beginning of treatment. Assessments are used to evaluate the effectiveness of specific interventions used in the course of a series of treatments, as well as patients' progress toward rehabilitation goals independent of treatment. This must be expected to be true for cognitive assessment as much as for more traditional types.

Evaluation of treatment effectiveness is potentially a special application of any clinical assessment approach. In this application there are specific issues that play themselves out differently in the clinical setting as opposed to the research laboratory. In the context of basic research, three issues to be addressed to assess whether an intervention is effective are: 1) Does the treatment work better than no treatment at all? 2) Does one particular treatment do more than alternative treatments? 3) What are the actual (as opposed to theoretical or putative) mechanisms by which the treatment exerts its effects? In the context of evaluating the progress of individual patients, the issues are different: 1) Has the patient improved or not? 2) Are the improvements continuously dependent on some situational factor (e.g., a prosthetic environment), or have they gained some functional autonomy? 3) Do the improvements really contribute to any meaningful change in the patient's personal or social functioning or quality of life?

It seems certain that in the future researchers and clinicians will be using cognitive assessment to evaluate the outcome of various treatments, and they will be using various other outcome measures to evaluate the effects of cognitive therapy. It will be important for everyone to remember that the relevant questions are different in the clinical and laboratory contexts. Regardless of research findings, cognitive technology will be successful in the clinical setting only if it can successfully address the clinician's concerns. On the other hand, much of the promise of cognitive assessment technology lies in the possibility that it will elucidate the mechanisms of various intervention approaches, leading to development of increasingly efficient techniques.

The question was raised whether cognitive assessment data can instruct group leaders about the learning style of the person assessed, so that material can be presented and taught more effectively. The question suggests a convergence of basic research and clinical application concerns about the mechanisms of treatment effects. Possibly, factors analogous to "learning style" can be assessed clinically, and the resulting information can be used to fine-tune learning-based treatment. It was agreed that this application could turn out to be useful. However, current research is a long way from validating any interpretive approach that could perform such a role. As a caution against premature clinical application of complex and poorly understood cognitive data, it was pointed out that the therapist's expectation of a person's performance in a group is known to be an important variable in performance. An influence of expectations based on invalid interpretation of cognitive assessment data would be most undesirable.

This interpretive caveat led to more general discussion of interpretive problems. Cognitive performance, whether in laboratory tasks, formal in vivo assessments, or group therapy and skills training, is affected by a host of variables. "Motivation" to engage in the task is a major source of interpretive confusion. In the long term, a complete understanding of cognitive functioning must incorporate motivation, possibly by way of an understanding of the relationship between cognition and emotion. Meanwhile, cognitive performance needs to be assessed in many different situations across which motivation and interest vary. Legitimate clinical techniques for manipulating motivation, such as token economy, may turn out to be crucial adjuncts to any assessment of cognitive functioning, especially in the most severely disordered patients.

The tension and impatience associated with different perspectives and professional backgrounds were apparent at the conference as assessment issues were discussed. The differences between questions important in research and questions important in clinical application clearly contributed to the tension. In addition, different theoretical and professional backgrounds seemed associated with different priorities about what kind of information is to be expected from clinical assessment. For some, molecular processes such as attention and memory are of paramount importance. For others, the molar cognitive processes that can be most directly associated with functional abilities (such as doing the laundry or balancing a checking account) must take precedence. What implicitly emerged from this discussion was that for cognitive assessment to be accepted by everyone, a network of validating functional relationships will have to evolve, uniting the foci of interest of various rehabilitation professionals. If neuropsychological data is to be accepted as useful by therapists, it will have to be shown that deficits in attention and memory are truly core problems that affect a diversity of functional impairments. If molar cognitive analyses of skill performance are to be accepted as scientifically legitimate, they will have to be consistent with what is known about the effects of psychopathology on more basic cognitive functions. With a full and shared understanding of these relationships, the relative importance of one or another focus in assessment becomes an administrative issue. Depending on the purpose of a specific treatment intervention or the mission of a particular rehabilitation program, more emphasis would be expected on one focus than on another.

A twist in the discussion of the usefulness of cognitive assessments was the question of whether assessments always need to eventuate in a specific intervention or treatment approach to improve the identified deficits. On the one hand, assessments that do not directly indicate therapeutic solutions may have questionable usefulness in a functionally oriented rehabilitation program. On the other hand, restricting assessments to problems for which there are currently known or available treatments could lead to distorted views of the comprehensiveness and effectiveness of programs, and could stifle research on new treatment approaches. This may be another dilemma whose resolution lies in an administrative domain. The scope and nature of assessment data available to a service program should follow from a fully articulated and context-sensitive understanding of that program's mission in the mental health system.

In general, the discussion of cognitive assessment issues revealed consensus that such information is potentially useful in psychiatric rehabilitation. Differences of opinion revolved around the appropriate scope of assessment, the degree to which functional utility should guide development of assessment packages, and the relationship between research and application priorities. The resolution of these disagreements appears to lie as much in administrative considerations about the role of specific programs in the larger mental health system as in technical considerations about cognitive assessment per se. For that reason, discussion of assessment issues often led to discussion about the role of rehabilitation in the larger mental health system.

The Nature of Mental Health Systems

Enthusiasm among the conference participants for the promise of cognitive technology was tempered by concerns about the difficulty with which mental health systems adopt any new technology. The sources of this difficulty identified by various discussants included: 1) the lack of common models among agencies within service systems; 2) disincentives, which operate on entire systems, as well as individuals within the system, to discourage any innovation or change; 3) lack of funds sufficient to support the costs of retooling; 4) rivalries and turf battles between professions; 5) distrust between the researchers who develop new technologies and the clinicians who use them; 6) the methodological difficulty of demonstrating that any approach to assessment and treatment is more cost-effective than any other.

Many of these problems are interdependent. In that sense, collaboration emerged as a strategic approach to solutions. Greater collaboration between clinicians and researchers could generally improve the immediate clinical relevance of cognitive technology research, giving clinicians more input into the research planning process and researchers more exposure to practical problems. Greater collaboration between the various mental health disciplines could facilitate development of common language and construct systems, overcoming, for example, some of the confusion that was evident in discussions of clinical assessment issues. This would in turn clarify the special contributions of the various disciplines; it is lack of consensus about the uniqueness of those contributions that fuels interdisciplinary disputes. Greater collaboration between service provision agencies and research institutions could facilitate identification of common interests and goals, leading to joint pursuit of federal funds for system-wide outcome research.

Mental health service systems are increasingly data-driven. Since the rehabilitation approach is highly empirical, this should facilitate the eventual adoption of cognitive technologies. However, this possibility also reintroduces the conflict between basic research and application priorities. The data that drive mental health systems concern the costs of specific services, as delivered in the system's own environment, compared with the individual and community-wide benefits of the services. The data that drive cognitive research concern the mechanistic effects of treatment, delivered in a highly contrived environment, without direct regard for costs or benefits. Collaboration will therefore be successful only to the degree that clinicians and administrators are willing to invest in at least some expenses that will not necessarily yield cost-effective results, and to the degree that researchers are willing to compromise on laboratory control to protect the pristine interpretability of their results.

The point was made in various ways that mental health systems are not purely data-driven. Any mental health administrator must weigh cost-effectiveness considerations against a multiplicity of political and social policy factors. The complexities of state and federal health care reimbursement systems are among these, although it may be difficult to distinguish the politics from the economics of these systems. In the private sector, such systems are often the chief battleground for interprofessional struggles. Policy set for the private sector can affect public sector economics. Resolution of these struggles may therefore have profound effects on how or even whether cognitive technology is eventually adopted in mental health service systems.

Ethical Issues

Ethical concerns ranged from the effects of labeling individuals based on the outcome of assessments to the role of government in the "prescription" of interventions. The concerns added layers of complexity to already complex issues. For example, questions about the extent to which a governmental overseer of public services can or should influence the types of interventions used lead to: What happens when what is better for the consumer is not what is better for a financially constrained government? Is there consensus within the scientific community on the effectiveness of technology, a consensus that can guide administrative policy? Can the public expect clinical work to reflect state-of-the-art technology? Should administrators depend on the standards and judgments of regulatory agencies and accrediting commissions? If so, which ones? And should accreditation address service process or content?

It was suggested that the problem of labeling, of defining an individual in terms of a disability or impairment, must be addressed by assessing the whole person, considering the individual's strengths and vulnerabilities at multiple levels. Such a broad basis reduces the risk of stigmatizing labels and it enhances clinical services, since in fact it is the whole person who is experiencing rehabilitation. The common language of a service system can be more or less prone to stigmatization, and this is perhaps one of the risks of developing common languages. It was also noted, however, that any label is only as good or bad as its use (or abuse) in a service system. Faultless terminology is no substitute for ethically sensitive and technologically sophisticated personnel. Both are probably necessary for adequately descriptive yet stigma-free clinical communication.

Professional and Training Issues

If any one issue can predictably generate heat without light in a group with multiple professional representation, it is the issue of training—who should be trained to do what. While a bit of momentary heat was generated early in the conference, the issues of training and professional purview, raised periodically throughout the conference, became ones in which professional differences were appreciated more than disdained.

The medical model as a basis of professional training was mentioned only briefly. This is somewhat surprising, inasmuch as the value and even legitimacy of that model has been a focus of debate in psychopathology and mental health. It is possible that the various arguments associated with this debate have become so familiar that few are interested in reviewing them yet again. Another possibility is that the term "medical model" has been used to refer to so many different things that its meaning is too ambiguous to spawn debate. The term refers sometimes to biomedical illness-based conceptualizations of behavior problems, sometimes to health care structures wherein physicians occupy primary and hegemonic administrative positions, and sometimes to a hypothetical-deductive approach to clinical problem solving that seems indistinguishable from general descriptions of the scientific method. In this context, the question of whether any discipline's training is rooted in "the medical model" or alternative models seems not to lead directly to clarification of interprofessional issues.

The point was made that interprofessional rivalry is anathema to the concept of rehabilitation, because the multiplicity of technologies involved demands the involvement of a number of highly and specially trained professionals. Basic training within the various mental health disciplines does not address psychiatric rehabilitation sufficiently. The bulk of training in psychiatric rehabilitation takes place after the professional degree has been obtained, and it takes place in an interdisciplinary environment. While there are narrow bands of professional purview, much of psychiatric rehabilitation is a wide field in which professionals must work on a collaborative bases.

Just as collaboration was identified as vital to the improvement of services and service delivery within the system, so collaboration is vital in addressing training needs. The fact that professions need each other in order to get the work done was stated in various ways. Nevertheless, it remained unclear in the course of the discussion how deep is the understanding and appreciation of the breadth and depth of training in the various disciplines. In any case, interprofessional rivalries did not inhibit the conference. Differing perspectives, sometimes identifiable as stemming from disciplinary and professional differences, resulted in more lively discussion.

The emerging role of computers in cognitive assessment and treatment inspired a comment that the human qualities of clinical activities must not be neglected. This is not simply a plea for humanistic values, but a reminder that interpersonal transactions are known to be an important source of psychotherapeutic effects. There is no reason to believe that the same is not true for cognitive therapy effects. Careful research is needed to clarify which kinds of assessment and treatment require the element of interaction between patient and human clinician. What we learn from this research must inform training strategies for all mental health disciplines, perhaps some in different ways than others.

Conclusion

The conference discussions revealed areas in which there appears to be a high degree of agreement. One concerns the need for and usefulness of cognitive assessment in rehabilitation, and the role of assessment in measuring the effectiveness of treatment and elucidating its mechanisms.

A second area of agreement was the desire for and need for greater collaboration within the service delivery system and among the mental health disciplines. This collaboration would enhance the possibility of developing a common language and shared concepts. The need for interdisciplinary cooperation and appreciation was well accepted, and was suggested as a basis for developing innovative funding strategies as well as service programs.

The importance of empiricism and cost-effectiveness analysis was never directly challenged. However, there was no clear consensus about whether scientific validity should be the ultimate criterion in service planning, nor about how it should be translated into administrative policy.

It became clear that clinicians are often not familiar with the history of research and theory that is the foundation for cognitive assessments. Whether a greater familiarity, or at least a greater awareness, would encourage a more helpful perspective for clinicians is not known. Without this perspective, the desire for clinical applications from basic research tends to lead to frustration for both clinicians and researchers.

As in many town meetings, it seems premature to vote on what is right or wrong, or on what to do or not to do. The conference became a time to share perspectives, smoke out and question implicit assumptions, and entertain new ideas to approach old questions.

THE CONTRIBUTORS

Claudia Kay Allen, MA, OTR, FAOTA, is a clinical associate professor in the Department of Occupational Therapy and the Department of Psychiatry and Behavioral Sciences, University of Southern California.

M. T. Appelo is a lecturer in the Department of Clinical Psychology, University of Gröningen, and a clinical psychologist at the "Licht en Kracht" Psychiatric Hospital, Assen, The Netherlands.

Peter G. Beeson, PH.D, is the director of planning, Nebraska Department of Public Institutions, and a graduate lecturer in the departments of sociology and social work, University of Nebraska.

R. J. van den Bosch, PH.D, is a professor of psychiatry, University of Gröningen, The Netherlands.

Mark DeKraai, JD, PH.D, is a mental health systems planner and policy analyst in the Nebraska Department of Public Institutions.

Richard C. Erickson, PH.D, is a staff psychologist at the Seattle Veterans Administration Medical Center and an associate professor of psychiatry and behavioral sciences, University of Washington Medical School.

Susan B. Fine, MA, OTR, FAOTA, is an assistant clinical professor in the College of Health-related Professions, State University of New York Health Science Center; a senior lecturer in therapeutic activities, Department of Psychiatry, Cornell Medical College; and director of therapeutic activities at Payne Whitney Clinic, New York Hospital – Cornell Medical Center.

Mark van der Gaag, PH.D, is a clinical psychologist in the Department of Psychiatry, University of Leiden, and at the "Endegeest" Psychiatric Hospital, Oegstgeest, The Netherlands.

Joel O. Goldberg, PH.D, is an assistant professor in the Department of Psychiatry, McMaster University, and clinical director of the Hamilton program for schizophrenia, Hamilton, Ontario.

Michael F. Green, PH.D, is an assistant research professor in the Department of Psychiatry and Biobehavioral Sciences, Neuropsychiatric Institute, University of California–Los Angeles, and co-director of the neuropsychology program at the Camarillo Neuropsychiatric Institute.

Robert K. Heinssen, PH.D, is chief of behavior therapy, Chestnut Lodge Hospital, Rockville, Maryland.

Robert S. Kern, PH.D, is a postdoctoral fellow in the neuropsychology program of the Camarillo Neuropsychiatric Institute.

J. W. Louwerens, MD, is a psychiatrist in the Department of Psychiatry, University of Gröningen, and the "Licht en Kracht" Psychiatric Hospital, Assen, The Netherlands.

Peter A. Magaro, PH.D, is a professor of psychology and psychiatry, Cornell Medical Center, and director of research for the National Association on Drug Abuse Problems, Inc.

Robert L. Schalock, PH.D, is the chairperson in the Department of Psychology, Hastings College, and an adjunct research professor of medical psychology, University of Nebraska Medical Center.

C. J. Slooff, PH.D, is a clinical psychologist in the Department of Psychiatry, University of Gröningen, and the "Licht en Kracht" Psychiatric Hospital, Assen, The Netherlands.

Mary Sullivan, MSW, CMSW, is a clinical assistant professor in the Department of Psychology, University of Nebraska–Lincoln, and director of the extended care unit, Lincoln Regional Center, Lincoln, Nebraska.

William D. Spaulding, PH.D, is a professor of psychology at the University of Nebraska–Lincoln.

Brian K. Victor, MA, is a research assistant at Chestnut Lodge Hospital, Rockville, Maryland.

F. M. J. Woonings, MD, is a psychiatrist at the "Licht en Kracht" Psychiatric Hospital, Assen, The Netherlands.

Index